The Most Decadent Diet Ever!

The MOST DECADENT DIET *Ever!*

Devin Alexander

with a Foreword by Kate Geagan, MS, RD, founder of IT Nutrition, LLC

PHOTOGRAPHY BY THERESA RAFFETTO

BROADWAY BOOKS · NEW YORK

BROADWAY

PUBLISHED BY BROADWAY BOOKS

Copyright © 2008 by Devin Alexander

All Rights Reserved

Published in the United States by Broadway
Books, an imprint of The Doubleday Broadway
Publishing Group, a division of Random House,
Inc., New York.

www.broadwaybooks.com

BROADWAY BOOKS and its logo,
a letter B bisected on the diagonal,
are trademarks of Random House, Inc.

Book design by Elizabeth Rendfleisch

Library of Congress Cataloging-in-Publication
Data

Alexander, Devin.
    The Most decadent diet ever! / by Devin
Alexander; photography by Theresa Raffetto.
—1st ed.
        p.   cm.
    Includes index.
1. Reducing diets—Recipes. I. Title.
    RM222.2.A3794 2008
    641.5'635—dc22
2007037652

ISBN 978-0-7679-2881-6

PRINTED IN THE UNITED STATES OF AMERICA

10 9 8 7 6 5 4 3 2 1

First Edition

This book is dedicated
to my mother, Toni Simone,
who saw me as
"Pretty (Plus)" even when
I was at my heaviest.

My career has made her life
a little less private than
she'd like it to be, yet she's
still the best support
a girl could have.

Mom, you're the best!

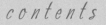

contents

As a registered dietitian and nutrition expert with a successful corporate wellness practice, I've worked with thousands to help them lose weight, manage chronic disease, and improve their health through diet. That's how I know that Devin's story is the story of millions of Americans who struggle with weight and want a healthy way to eat *they can stick with* that will lead to weight loss.

Americans have expanding waistlines and a growing obsession with quick fixes. Chronic diseases are at an all-time high. And surveys prove that most Americans know what they should be eating. They just don't know *how*.

The research is clear: To see long-term weight loss and health improvements, a healthy way of eating must become a lifestyle, not a short-term diet. This new way must be tasty and must include healthy versions of the foods people crave—all while meeting calorie and nutrient goals.

Meet Devin Alexander, your new best friend! With her honest, straightforward, and humorous approach, Devin is just what the doctor (and dietitian) ordered! When you hear her personal story and cooking philosophy, when you see how this has brought her tremendous, long-term success, you'll discover that this is *not* a diet book at all, but a sound approach to a new lifestyle of joy, delight in food, and freedom from weight cycling. As any dietitian or health profession will tell you, this is precisely the type of success on which you can model your own healthier, slimmer future.

Devin's easy eating plan demonstrates how to manage cravings while committing to health priorities. Devin *gets* it—she's been there with us—experiencing late-night cravings and anxious moments stepping on the scale and hoping for a miracle rather than an accurate reflection of how you've behaved all week. With *The Most Decadent Diet Ever!*, Devin will be with you as you make these changes—a new best friend (who doubles as a gastronomic goddess) with a sound handle on nutrition and health.

No matter your cooking skills, Devin shows you easy ways to reinvent decadent flavors, using common ingredients and calorie-appropriate portion sizes—without giving up foods you enjoy. And even if you are currently finding success with another eating style, this book is a great companion on those inevitable days when you're dying for some comfort food, when you're looking for a fun change of pace without loading up on calories, saturated fat, and salt, or even when you want something decadent on hand for company but don't want to blow the plan you're on because it's working well for you. Devin helps keep life flexible.

My career is built on a desire to help people understand what and how they should eat for optimum health. Devin's book is an invaluable tool because it offers a path for people who want to keep eating their favorites, with fewer calories and sound nutritional principles. *The Most Decadent Diet Ever!* shows you how to make all foods fit into a healthy eating plan that can be followed for life. Thankfully, Devin knows that life is just sweeter with chocolate!

I am excited and honored to support Devin in her quest to shrink America's waistline one delicious bite at a time. With her helpful tips, outstanding recipes, thoughtful nutritional approach, and personal track record of long-term weight maintenance, Devin is living proof that we can have our cake and eat it too.   —Kate Geagan, MS, RD, founder of IT Nutrition

preface

LET'S FACE IT, IF YOU FOLLOW A DIET, ANY DIET, IT WILL WORK. You *will* lose weight. But the problem is that time goes by and cravings grow, and if you're at all like me, you just can't stick to a diet. In fact, diets are likely to make you fatter or less healthy. The cycle goes something like this. You start the diet, you stick to it for a while (the amount of time "a while" comprises tends to be inversely proportional to the number of years you've already been "dieting"), and then you eat something "bad." That causes you to eat something else "bad" to the extent that you're no longer on the diet. So you declare that you'll start a new diet (or maybe the same diet) on Monday or next week or on January 1. But this creates the need to eat everything in sight that you might ever miss in the meantime . . . just in case. Sound familiar? That was my cycle for the eight years that I went from chubby to obese before starting my journey to *The Most Decadent Diet Ever!*

The Most Decadent Diet Ever! is not actually a diet in the sense of a follow-it-to-the-letter-type deprivation diet. It's a diet in the sense of a "way of eating." It's a lifestyle that affords you (and has afforded me!) tons of freedom. Though at first glance it may not appear that way, rest assured it is.

The collection of recipes in this book is in no way meant to constitute your entire eating regimen. That would be too limiting for anyone, as any collection of only 125-plus recipes would be. They're merely some of the most decadent dishes you may find yourself craving that you likely feel you "cannot" or "should not" eat when trying to be healthy. They can be used in many ways: as the basis for creating your own personal "diet" as outlined in this book; as a way to add some otherwise "off-limits" foods back into a traditional diet with which you're already succeeding; as the first step for those desperately needing a healthier lifestyle who just plain don't like "diet food"; or as a little slice of heaven for those who have already achieved maximum health but miss some of their favorites.

The recipes were carefully and laboriously constructed to be precisely 100, 200, 300, 400, or 500 calories (within 10 calories) to make it easy for you to keep track of what and how you're eating without requiring a calculator. The key thing to remember is that *The Most Decadent Diet Ever!* whether you choose to use it as a cookbook or a calorie-counting diet, is about freedom, not deprivation. And regardless of how you choose to use this book the day you pick it up, my hope is that eventually you stop counting calories forever (as I have) and just loosely adopt this plan in a way you can follow long-term, loving every minute of it.

THE MOST DECADENT DIET EVER! IS "THE SECRET" OF FOOD

By now, whether you've seen or read "The Secret," we've all heard about it. What you visualize, what you imagine, is what you create. When I was a teen, I was desperate to lose weight, so I put so much negative energy into trying to lose it. I was obsessed and had nightmares. I was chronically dieting and I kept getting fatter.

By my twenties I was still obsessed with food, but I figured out how to get thin by re-creating my favorite dishes. Sadly, I succumbed to the pressures of living near Hollywood and spent years eating bland salads and tons of rabbit food and became too thin for my body type.

Then, in my mid- to late twenties, I finally decided that food isn't the enemy. It is something that I have a deep love and affinity for. It's something that I enjoy (probably more than many), so it should be my friend.

I started being creative with food. And I made a conscious decision never to go on a diet again. As a result, for over sixteen years, my weight has fluctuated only within seven pounds. Why? I've found "The Secret" of food.

When I gave up dieting and stopped labeling my favorites like chocolate and burgers "bad," I was happier and more satisfied. If I started craving chocolate, I knew I could have it. I just had to cook it a little differently from most of those store-bought cakes and cookies. I started imagining rich, warm, flourless deep chocolate cakes (see Chocolate Not-Only-in-Your-Dreams Cake, page 210), fettuccine Alfredo (see Fettu-Skinny Alfredo, page 104), and drippy burgers (see BBQ Bacon Cheeseburger, page 57; Blue Cheese Mushroom Burger, page 55; etc.), and I saw myself enjoying them guilt free.

I was suddenly able to vacation with friends (I used to turn down trips in fear that I couldn't get food I needed to stay thin) and would often cook or end up enjoying getting everyone involved in cooking as a group on the trips. And that led to greater popularity and less isolation (so often people eat simply because they're lonely). I stopped worrying about every little thing I put in my mouth. I stopped worrying about what I would do if I showed up at a boyfriend's mother's house and they didn't have healthy food. I stopped worrying about what I'd eat at a business lunch. None of it would destroy my diet because I wasn't on one. I ate healthy food as much as possible, and if I had to eat one meal that was a little more fattening, it was suddenly no big deal, because I was able to see it as one fattening meal, not the end of a diet.

And once I started enjoying the healthier versions, I didn't want the fattening ones. There were no longer debates going on in my head when I was supposed to be paying attention to conversations. I knew that I truly didn't want the 746-calorie, 38-grams-of-fat slice of choc-olate layer cake at dinner, because I could make one (see Dark Chocolate Layer Cake with Chocolate Buttercream Frosting, page 208) with 294 calories and 6 grams of fat that I could enjoy guilt free.

DESPERATE TIMES REQUIRE DEVIN'S MEASURES

When I was desperate to lose weight, I went to a nutritionist. I think I secretly (or not so secretly) hoped that she was going to tell me that I had some sort of medical reason for being overweight. But the truth was: I love(d) food.

Instead of telling me that I could take a few more B vitamins and my metabolism would suddenly kick in (allowing me to eat chocolate fudge cake whenever I wanted, which was . . . well, always), she had the nerve to suggest that I should eat baked chicken, baked potatoes, and steamed broccoli as the mainstay of my diet. Then she sat there and described in detail just how tasty she found apples to be.

In retrospect, it's kind of funny. I know, as most Americans do, what I "should" be eating. And in the perfect world, there would be no such thing as sugar, no such thing as white flour, and no such thing as cravings. But, particularly for some of us, there are. I truly believe that some of us are just wired in a way that we crave foods. So although I wholeheartedly and adamantly assert that all of our diets "should" be primarily composed of lean proteins, whole grains, fruits, and plenty of fresh (and dare I even say "organic" and "local"?) veggies, all prepared with as little sodium as possible, it's just not realistic for some of us to eat that way.

I tried. I struggled. I obsessed. I even gave up sugar and white flour for years and found a weight-loss club to muscle through sticking to it. And I was miserable. I was also a heck of a lot less productive than I am today because I wasted so much time hashing and rehashing my own and others' weight-loss woes.

When I finally let go of all of the negativity and decided that I would never go on another diet, I lost the weight. If I craved chocolate cake, I'd figure out a way to make a healthier one. If I craved rigatoni with meat sauce, I'd focus my energies in the kitchen. If I craved a sausage sandwich, I'd rip apart my favorite one as many times as it would take to re-create those flavors. And suddenly, I never had to diet again.

acknowledgments

I'm extremely blessed to be surrounded by such a hugely professional, committed group of people—so much so that my friends started calling them "Team Devin":

To the whole crew at Broadway: my accomplished editor, Jennifer Josephy, and art director and designer, Elizabeth Rendfleisch. To Tammy Blake, ace publicist, and Lindsay Gordon, and to Catherine Pollock and Julie Sills in marketing. To Jennifer's assistant, Stephanie Bowen. They've made this process so exciting.

To my right-hand gal and assistant recipe developer, Stephanie Farrell, and my assistants and recipe testers, Lindsey Dietsch and Erin Sayers, who are utter godsends. And to Heather Haque, who has been assisting with my ventures since college.

To my manager, Julie Carson May, and publicist, Mary Lengle, who astound me every day, and whom I'm lucky enough to also call friends. And to Matt Krimmer, attorney extraordinaire.

To the extremely talented Deborah Feingold, who made the cover shoot an absolute blast. And to Jeff Gautier, hair and makeup ultra-wizard.

To my friends John Baker, Corbin Bell, Adrian Borden, Christine Boyer, Rasha Chapman, Alyssa Devore, Tony Dimond, Jim Eber, Steve Farrell, Kelly Frazier, Gail Gillman, Tas Haque, Pattianna Harootian, Grace Kung, Sandy Levin, Michelle Miller, Jamie Nehasil, Chris Nielsen, Nick Nunez, Kristine Oller, Stephanie Perfect, Amanda Philipson, Lara Scatamacchia, Alex Scott, Dawn Sostrin, Rita and Josh Sostrin, Jerry Whitworth, Apollo Yiamouyiannis, and Julieann Chism Zvik, for lending their support and taste buds.

To Kate Geagan, MS, RD, who generously lent her expertise.

To Theresa Raffetto and food stylist Victoria Granof, who made the food jump off the pages.

To the folks at *The Biggest Loser,* especially Mark Koops, J. D. Roth, Todd A. Nelson, Dave Broome, Chad Bennett, and, of course, Ben Silverman, who have continually welcomed me into their world.

To Meyer Corporation, for graciously keeping me well stocked with my favorite cookware (Infinite Circulon) to develop the recipes with and to use on my shows. And to Heinz and Weight Watchers Smart Ones, who fill my freezer with plenty of the most decadent frozen entrées for those times when I just don't have time to cook.

And last, but not least, to my entire family, led by my dad and his mantra, "Keep on keeping on," with special thanks to my sister, Leslie, for always being younger and wiser.

READY, SET, GO HEALTHY

So you're ready to start using *The Most Decadent Diet Ever!* and you need to know how it works. Here are your options:

Option 1: You're Already Following a Diet

If you've already found success on a particular diet plan and you are enjoying the process of losing weight or staying fit, congratulations. That's quite a feat. In that case, simply flip through the pages to find recipes that complement that diet. Then jump right in using those recipes.

Option 2: You're Not Following a Diet, but You Need to Get Healthier, and You Have No Desire to Count Calories Ever

No problem. Simply start cooking dishes from this book that are similar to what you're eating. Also, stick to portions that are no bigger than portions you are currently eating. If you know you're eating too much, start by making them slightly smaller than your present ones. Also, always include plenty of fresh fruits and veggies in your diet. The fiber will help fill you and also help your body process foods better and get the vitamins and minerals it craves.

When calculating portions, I always try to eat as follows (this is a general set of rules):

Protein: I eat about 4 ounces of lean meat, poultry, or seafood at each meal (unless a dish is providing protein from another source also, such as light cheese; then it might be a bit less):

- Boneless, skinless chicken breast, or ground chicken breast
- Boneless, skinless turkey breast, or ground turkey breast
- Pork tenderloin
- 96% lean ground beef
- Top round steak
- Other very lean meats
- Four large egg whites
- Seafood

Four ounces is about the size of a deck of cards or the size of my palm. Guys, who may want to eat 6 ounces, can also use their palms as a guide for that.

Veggies: I eat as many low-starch vegetables (e.g., broccoli, bell peppers, etc.) as I want, and recommend you do the same—that is, if you're just eating plain veggies. If they're decadent veggies, be wary of the added fats. Though my recipes are much lower in fat and calories than the traditional versions, you don't want to eat goat cheese every time you eat a veggie.

Starchy or Sugary Carbohydrates: At each large meal, I try to eat either a large piece of fruit or about $1/2$ to 1 cup (in the case of pasta) of whole grains or potatoes:

- Brown rice
- Whole-grain pilaf
- A whole-grain bun
- Two slices of whole-grain bread (about 70 calories each, or 1 slice if more caloric)
- A low-fat, whole-grain tortilla (110–130 calories)
- Whole-grain or fiber-enriched pasta
- Sweet potatoes
- Potatoes (They're actually vegetables, but listed here because they're high in starch.)

Those are my mainstays at most meals. Since I love chocolate, if I want chocolate, I try to eat the lean protein and plenty of veggies or salad, then add in a dessert (or an alcoholic beverage).

Fat: I try to keep my fats to a minimum. At each meal, I get a bit of fat in my diet from either a touch of cheese, a little bit of extra virgin olive oil, or some lower-fat or light mayo.

Frequency: I eat about five times per day. It keeps me from ever being famished and thus needing to grab the first thing in front of me. And though many diets tell you not to eat past 6 P.M., I've found this does not work for me. True, you don't want to go to bed on a full stomach (or even a half-full stomach), but I do like a couple of hundred calories within two hours of bed. Think about it. If you stop eating at 6 P.M., and don't go to bed until 10, then wake up at 6 A.M., you've gone twelve hours

without fueling your body at all. That just doesn't work for me or my body.

My five meals per day have roughly 300–400 calories each. When I say *meals*, I don't differentiate between meals and snacks. It's all food and it's all great. If I've had a meal that's a little larger (maybe in the 500-calorie range, like the Sweet-and-Sour Chicken Bowl, page 147), I have a smaller meal (a snack like Tiny Tacos, page 193, with only about 200). And if I'm going to eat a large dessert with 300 calories (such as Dark Chocolate Layer Cake with Chocolate Buttercream Frosting, page 208), then I just eat that as a meal (the four other meals that day would contain many more nutrients).

Now, if I told you that you wouldn't have to count calories, why have I thrown all of these numbers at you? The idea is that you use the amounts of protein, carbohydrates, and so on, given as a general guide. Then your meals will fall into those general ranges as long as you're not adding too much fat to them. For instance, say you want a Western Skinny Scramble (page 40) for breakfast one morning. That's 200 calories. It gives you lean protein (four egg whites) and some veggies. So then you can add in your carbs as directed. If you like to eat a bit more at breakfast, add a 200-calorie option like two Chocolate Chip Pancakes (page 23) or a Banana Colada Smoothie (page 52).

If you want just a 100-calorie option, because you're more of an afternoon snacker like I am, have one pancake or half of the smoothie, or maybe indulge in two Banana-Coconut Mini-Muffins (page 48) after your omelet. Then for lunch, when you're craving the Chicken Enchilasagna (page 134), you'll also be set. If you select the 400-calorie option, you'll get just over 4 ounces of lean protein from the chicken. You'll be eating two corn tortillas (about 120 calories' worth of starchy carbohydrates), and the tomatoes from the sauce provide a little bit toward your veggie quotient.

The meals are all designed to loosely follow the preceding guidelines. After a little review, you can be a pro at decadent eating without consequences whether you're eating meals from this book, creating other favorites on your own, or joining your boss for a business lunch and need to order from a menu.

Option 3: A Loved One Is Overweight and You're Worried about Him or Her

This one is easy. Simply copy a few recipes for his or her favorite dishes from the book. Hide the book and start cooking from the pages. He or she will never know the difference, and you'll be doing him or her a huge favor.

Option 4: Nothing Has Ever Worked and You Need the Structure to Start a Plan That Will Work!

Though it is my goal for everyone eventually to move toward Option 2 (not counting calories), sometimes it's safer and easier to follow a plan to the letter, particularly if you are new to healthier eating. I used to count calories when I first created *The Most Decadent Diet Ever!* for myself. Now I don't have to. There's nothing wrong with following a plan, and I strongly encourage it if it's comfortable for you. Over time, though, you'll realize that the more freedom you find, the easier it will be to enjoy living a healthy lifestyle forever!

GETTING STARTED

So let's get started on *The Most Decadent Diet Ever!* You'll be happy to know that it's very simple. Not only can you easily use recipes from this book in conjunction with fresh fruits, veggies, etc., but you can supplement them with meals that you need to eat out, meals from the frozen foods aisle (which can be lifesavers when you're insanely busy), or the plethora of 100-calorie-portion packs that are suddenly prevalent throughout grocery stores.

First you need to figure out how many calories you need to consume to reach or maintain a healthy weight. That depends on several factors, including your height, weight, age, gender, and activity level. While a visit to a registered dietitian may be your best bet to determine your precise caloric needs based on your goals, there are many reputable Web sites with free online "calorie calculators" that can help you determine your own specific calorie needs. You punch in a few quick numbers and voilà!—a personalized calorie guide. "The key is to be sure to choose a calculator that is found on the site of a reputable, science-based institution, as opposed to a site that is connected to selling you a product," suggests Kate Geagan, MS, RD, a dietitian and nutrition expert. Two of her favorites include WebMD.com and the Baylor College of Medicine (www.bcm.edu/cnrc/caloriesneed.htm). If that's not an easy option either, the chart on the next page can serve as a rough guide for how many calories you need based on age, gender, and activity level.

ESTIMATED CALORIE REQUIREMENTS

These are the Estimated Energy Requirements included in the 2005 Dietary Guidelines for Americans, based on the Institute of Medicine's 2002 Dietary Reference Intakes Report.

Gender	Age (years)	Sedentary[a]	Moderately Active[b]	Active[c]
Female	4–8	1,200	1,400–1,600	1,400–1,800
	9–13	1,600	1,600–2,000	1,800–2,200
	14–18	1,800	2,000	2,400
	19–30	2,000	2,000–2,200	2,400
	31–50	1,800	2,000	2,200
	51+	1,600	1,800	2,000-2,200
Male	4–8	1,400	1,400–1,600	1,600–2,000
	9–13	1,800	1,800–2,200	2,000–2,600
	14–18	2,200	2,400–2,800	2,800–3,200
	19–30	2,400	2,600–2,800	3,000
	31–50	2,200	2,400–2,600	2,800–3,000
	51+	2,000	2,200–2,400	2,400–2,800

a Sedentary means a lifestyle that includes only the light physical activity associated with typical day-to-day life.

b Moderately active means a lifestyle that includes physical activity equivalent to walking about 1.5 to 3 miles per day at 3 to 4 miles per hour, in addition to the light physical activity associated with typical day-to-day life.

c Active means a lifestyle that includes physical activity equivalent to walking more than 3 miles per day at 3 to 4 miles per hour, in addition to the light physical activity associated with typical day-to-day life.

Public information from the U.S. Department of Health and Human Services

CALORIE CONSUMPTION FOR WEIGHT LOSS

While the above chart gives you an idea of your current calorie needs, if your goal is to lose weight you need to shake up this equation and start burning more calories than you consume. In order to lose one pound of body fat (because who wants to lose just water weight?), you need to create a deficit of 3,500 calories. The best way to lose fat, maintain lean muscle, and keep your metabolism moving is to plan to lose about 1 to 2 pounds per week; slashing calories too drastically can be counter-productive to your metabolism and energy levels (plus it's nearly impossible to stick with). This means you need to create about a 500-calorie deficit per day:

500 calories per day x 7 days = 3,500 calories, or 1 pound of fat

While you can do this by shaving 500 calories off your diet, an easier way (and one that's been shown to be much more successful in the long term) is to do it in a combination: Burn an extra 250 calories through exercise and shave

250 from your diet. "For most people, it's more appealing and doable to know that they can continue to have a few extra splurges in their diet if they are willing to move more," says Geagan. But do note that the American College of Sports Medicine (ACSM) recommends that calorie levels never drop below 1,200 calories per day for women or 1,800 calories per day for men, as anything below that is counterproductive to long-term weight-loss goals and may slow metabolism. If you are determined to go below this, please be sure to seek professional supervision. Remember, nothing in this book is meant to replace any advice from a certified medical professional.

DECIPHERING DECADENT DISKS

Now that you know how many calories you should be consuming, it's time to convert them to "Decadent Disks," which is as easy as can be:

1 Decadent Disk = 100 calories

So for every 100 calories you should be consuming, you eat 1 Decadent Disk's worth of food. That means that if you should consume 1,600 calories, you eat 16 Decadent Disks' worth of food every day. A 2-Decadent-Disk serving or portion would have approximately 200 calories.

CALORIES IN VERSUS CALORIES OUT

We've all heard it: if you increase activity and decrease the number of calories you consume (or both), you'll lose weight. And it's true. But there are also some other things to consider when choosing your meals and when following *The Most Decadent Diet Ever!*

- Eat at least 1½ cups of fruit and 2½ cups of veggies every day. (Visit www.mypyramid.gov for an exact amount based on your gender.)
- Get fiber in your diet; it not only fills you but also helps your body process foods.
- Complex carbohydrates such as whole grains keep you fuller longer than simple sugars.
- Eat many small meals throughout the day to keep your blood sugar regulated, hunger at bay, and your metabolism stimulated.
- Watch your sodium intake—you definitely don't want to overdo it.
- Drink at least eight glasses of water a day.
- Remember that the calories in alcoholic beverages count. Don't oversplurge.
- Don't consume large amounts of food before bedtime.
- The more active you are, the more weight you'll lose.
- Spicy food may help to stimulate your metabolism and immune system, so eating it can be a very good thing.
- Always read labels carefully when you're buying ingredients.
- Don't overindulge in sugar, particularly white sugar.
- Try to stick with lower-fat or light options of foods when the label tells you there's a calorie savings.
- Aim for 2 to 3 calcium-rich foods each day.
- Eat slowly—it takes twenty minutes for your stomach to tell your brain that you're full.
- Eat only until you feel lightly full, not stuffed.

The Most Decadent Diet Ever! Sample 7-Day Meal Plan—Based on 1,400 Calories per Day

	Day 1	Day 2	Day 3
Meal A	Vanilla, Chocolate, and Strawberry Breakfast Sundae	1 Breakfast Sausage Link 3 egg whites prepared with olive oil spray and topped with fresh salsa, (salsa optional) Potatoes O'Brien (1 Decadent Disk)	Chocolate Peanut Butter Breakfast "Pudding"
Meal B	Spinach Salad with Warm Bacon Dressing 3 ¹/₂ ounces Basic Grilled Chicken 1 cup fresh cherries	Chicken Pasta Salad (4 Decadent Disks)	Sexier Sausage and Pepper Sub
Meal C	Buffalo Wing Plate	Skinny Scampi 3/4 cup cooked protein-enriched pasta Roasted Ruby Tomatoes	Eggplant Parmesan 1 ¹/₂ cups fresh raspberries with 2 tablespoons fat-free whipped topping
Meal D	Chinese Pepper Steak ¹/₂ cup cooked brown rice 1 ¹/₂ cups steamed snow peas	Tiny Tacos (2 Decadent Disks)	Roast Beef with Horseradish Cream Parmesan-Garlic Mashed Potato Pancakes Sautéed Mushrooms au Vin
Meal E	2 Skinny-Mini Cherry-Topped Cheesecakes	Chocolate Not-Only-in-Your-Dreams Cake	Pumpkin Pie Bars (1 Decadent Disk) OR 4 ounces red wine
Nutrient Daily Total	115 g protein 185 g carbohydrates 28 g fat 9 g saturated fat 207 mg cholesterol 24 g fiber 2,186 mg sodium	110 g protein 176 g carbohydrates 32 g fat 8 g saturated fat 325 mg cholesterol 19 g fiber 1,918 mg sodium	92 g protein 194 g carbohydrates 31 g fat 9 g saturated fat 135 mg cholesterol 36 g fiber 2,143 mg sodium

Day 4	Day 5	Day 6	Day 7
1 Sinless Yet Sinful Sticky Bun Bacon Swiss Omelet (1 Decadent Disk)	Scrambled Eggs with Sautéed Shrimp 2 Banana-Coconut Mini-Muffins	Banana Colada Smoothie	Devin's Eggs On-the-Terrace Fruit Salad
1 3/4 cups sliced strawberries or 1 large apple Herbed Crab Salad (1 Decadent Disk)	Grilled Chicken Quesadilla	Gourmet Roast Beef Pocket Colorful Coleslaw	Muscles Meatloaf Sandwich
Potato Chip-Crusted Chicken Grilled Corn on the Cob	Blue Cheese Mushroom Burger	Mediterranean Layer Dip with Toasted Pita Triangles (2 Decadent Disks)	Fried Zucchini
Honey-Glazed Spiced Pork Tenderloin Horseradish Smashed Potatoes (1 Decadent Disk) Asparagus with Sherry Shallot Vinaigrette	Lemon-Thyme Chicken Kebabs Taboulied Couscous (1 Decadent Disk) 6 cups fresh spinach sautéed with 1/2 tsp olive oil and fresh garlic	Rigatoni with Meat Sauce	Sweet-and-Sour Chicken Bowl
Cinnamon Apple Yogurt Parfait	Roasted Pineapple à la Mode (1 Decadent Disk)	"Cleaner" Mud Pie	Godiva Brownie Sundae
97 g protein 185 g carbohydrates 35 g fat 11 g saturated fat 223 mg cholesterol 19 g fiber 1,901 mg sodium	142 g protein 142 g carbohydrates 35 g fat 11 g saturated fat 344 mg cholesterol 20 g fiber 2,373 mg sodium	83 g protein 218 g carbohydrates 30 g fat 11 g saturated fat 125 mg cholesterol 26 g fiber 2,239 mg sodium	97 g protein 199 g carbohydrates 26 g fat 5 g saturated fat 143 mg cholesterol 25 g fiber 2,240 mg sodium

PUTTING TOGETHER YOUR MENUS

Now that you know the number of Decadent Disks that make up your day, putting meals together is a cinch. To get the best balance possible and to learn the specifics about what has worked for me, please read Option 2 (page 1). Though you don't need to follow it to the letter, it is my experience and that's what I best know. But again, the most important thing is to befriend food; eat what you enjoy, while also getting plenty of fruits and veggies in your diet; and pick a way of "dieting" that you can stick to for life (and one that your doctor approves of, of course).

So here we are. It's time to start your journey! As you flip through this book and look at the pictures, I bet you're not going to want to "start tomorrow" or next week or even put it off until January 1. And with only a couple of bites, I'm sure you'll be ready to make a commitment . . . to you. Whether this is your first time wanting to eat a bit healthier or you've been dieting for years, you can do this!

The week of sample menus starting on page 6 is based on a 1,400-calorie intake. If you've decided to consume fewer calories, you can simply omit an item or two. If you, like me, require more calories, you can add portions or servings as needed to reach your desired calorie target. But remember: if you never follow this menu to the letter, that's okay. It's simply here to give you a sense of what great foods you can eat and how to put them together.

I tend to eat a bit less for breakfast, but am always in need of a late-afternoon energy boost, so I make sure to leave plenty of

calories for that time of day. You may love to start your day off with a big breakfast and then taper off through the day; that's okay too. These foods can be eaten in any order. The goal is to eat just as many Decadent Disks' worth of food as you (or your nutritionist) have allotted you, spacing them apart so you keep your metabolism kicked in.

Now if you're looking at this plan thinking, "Oh my God, I don't have time to make all of that," don't worry. Although most of the meals can be made easily in less than thirty minutes, I get that you may have a busy night. I often do too. If you don't have time to make the Stuffed Shells (page 102), simply buy a 300-calorie (3-Decadent-Disk) lasagna or any other healthy frozen entrée that appeals in that calorie range. If you don't love baking, you can skip the Sinless Yet Sinful Sticky Buns (page 49), and swap in any 2-Decadent-Disk breakfast item, such as the Banana Colada Smoothie (page 52) or a 200-calorie (2-Decadent-Disk) reduced-fat chocolate-chocolate-chip muffin from the freezer at your local grocery store. Or if you prefer your sweets at night, eat the sticky bun at night and have the Cinnamon Apple Yogurt Parfait (page 53) with the omelet at breakfast.

SERVINGS VERSUS PORTIONS

I've always wondered about people who can eat just a couple of bites of a dessert or two potato chips and actually feel satisfied. My mother is one of them and boy, do I wish she'd passed that gene on to me.

You'll notice that throughout the book, there are "portions" and "servings." A "serving" is a more standard, hearty amount of a dish. If you're sitting down to a meal and really want to be satiated, you'll find a serving to be the most realistic option. However, there are times, even for me, when a little bit (meaning about $\frac{1}{3}$ of a cup, in many cases) is enough to create a little freedom. That's where portions come in.

I eat portions (think of these as "freedom portions") of things like mashed potatoes and desserts often. For instance, suppose it's nighttime and I'm craving something a little bit sweet, but don't need a whole dessert. I just want "a little something." A 100-calorie (1-Decadent-Disk) portion gives me the freedom to have a great (yet small) dessert. Or if it's dinnertime and I want something a bit more substantial than just some London broil and salad, I have a portion (about $\frac{1}{3}$ cup) of mashed potatoes. One-third cup is a small scoop; I get the freedom to eat something decadent, but it's far from what your husband or dad with a healthy appetite would call a serving. The 100-calorie (1-Decadent-Disk) or even 200-calorie (2-Decadent-Disk) portions are great to keep you on track while satisfying cravings, yet leave you plenty of calories to fill up on the healthiest options when you're really watching carefully.

EAT, DRINK, AND BE MERRY

Good news: you don't have to give up alcohol on this plan. Again, though, moderation is key. A drink or two per week can easily be worked in. But be careful. Those calories add up quickly and they are, for the most part, empty calories. If you don't already know how many calories are in your favorite drink, it's helpful to find out.

When I'm going to be having a margarita or a Cosmo or another drink with sugar, I skip dessert that day, leaving enough calories for it. I eat more protein and veggies and then treat the drink as my carbs for the meal. But again, if you do this often, you'll be robbing yourself of essential nutrients that your body needs to feel great.

Make sure you account for any beverages in your diet and are knowledgeable about what you are drinking. Those calories count too. Anything can be worked into *The Most Decadent Diet Ever!* Just make sure that you are working them in and not ignoring them.

DON'T THROW SALT IN MY WOUNDS

Dietary guidelines suggest consuming less than 2,400 mg of sodium per day. Well, did you know that 4 ounces of the standard "healthy" turkey you buy at your local grocery store contains about 1,000 milligrams (mg) of sodium? Did you know that a typical 2-ounce link of breakfast sausage has about 551 mg? Did you know that two typical small (4-inch-diameter) pancakes have about 500 mg of sodium? Did you know that a couple of bites of lox contains about 567 mg? Or that $\frac{1}{4}$ cup of crumbled blue cheese has close to 400 mg of sodium? Did you know that a standard hamburger bun (3 $\frac{1}{2}$-inch diameter; white or whole-wheat) has about 206 mg of sodium, and a 6 $\frac{1}{2}$- to 7-inch flour tortilla often has about 330 mg? How about that 1 tablespoon of Dijon mustard has about 195 mg? Kind of daunting, isn't it, particularly since these are foods we love. But these are the foods we keep buying and the ones we keep craving, and, in some cases, even the ones we turn to when we're trying to eat healthy.

So I'm just going to say it: admittedly, some of the dishes in this book are much higher in sodium than I'd like them to be. I wrestled with this a lot. How do I bring folks the dishes they love, the ones they write to me about, in a healthier way without all of the sodium? Unfortunately, in some cases, I just can't cut the sodium as much as I'd like without sacrificing flavor.

If you look carefully, you'll notice that even among most of the dishes that are higher in sodium, the sodium count is still much lower than the traditional version of the dish you're used to eating. For example, we reduced the sodium in the Renovated Reuben Wrap (page 80) by about 20 percent as compared to a traditional Reuben of the same size, but as much as 75 percent over one that you'd typically be served.

What it comes down to is that if your doctor has told you to restrict your salt intake, listen to your doctor and be extremely mindful in following this plan or any plan. If, like me, you're simply trying to adopt a healthier lifestyle for you and your family, these dishes are *much* better than the "regular" versions. And if you crave a dish, and eating it will help you stick to a healthier "diet" in general, then I'm doing what I set out to do—provide lifelong alternatives, not extremes.

Just be wary of sodium as you plan your menus. Balance out your selections and eat higher-sodium dishes only when you're really craving them as opposed to using them as everyday staples. Steer clear of too many high-sodium dishes in any one day. And remember, eating plenty of fruits and veggies daily, in addition to watching your sodium, will help keep your blood pressure and heart healthy.

FLAVOR FIRST

As you flip through this book, you may notice that in some instances I use low-fat mayonnaise (3 grams of fat or less per serving) and in others I use light (a label meaning reduced by at least 50 percent of the fat or one third of the calories). In some dishes, I use brown rice, while in others I use white. In some dishes I use whole-grain oat flour or wheat flour, and in others I use white.

To me, flavor always comes first. So often the media reinforces the message that healthy food doesn't taste good. And then those same reporters or television hosts try my dishes and say, "How do you do that?" When I set out to re-create a dish, the process can take days, often even weeks. My assistants and I run test after test to find the best possible formula for optimum taste with the best health. Sometimes that means that after attempting to make a dish with oat flour, we return to white. Sometimes after using low-sodium instead of lower-sodium chicken broth, we realize that the dish goes from tasting delicious to tasting like bathwater (this is common with broth-based soups), and we resort to using a bit more sodium than desired. But in the end, we've compiled a "diet" book full of delicious alternatives just as good as, if not better than, the ones you're currently indulging in.

BUT I'M TOO BUSY . . .

I know, I know, we're all too busy to cook. Except that cooking can actually save you time. Cooking is like riding a bike. When you start it seems tough, but later it's a breeze. Even the grocery shopping becomes effortless when you learn to locate the ingredients you need.

I always say that I'd prefer twenty minutes in the kitchen over three hours on a stair-climber any day. If you consider how much time you'd have to spend in the gym to be healthy after eating so many restaurant dishes, cooking actually saves you time. Plus, if you're one of the millions visiting your doctor on a regular basis for high blood pressure, high cholesterol, lethargy, diabetes, sleep apnea, or one of the many other diseases that can be a direct result of unhealthy eating, you're not only wasting time, you're wasting money—money that could save you from working so much, thus freeing up even more time.

Plus, when you go out to lunch at work, you're spending a lot of money and tons of time. What if you were to make Roast Beef with Horseradish Cream (page 121) for your family's dinner, and then a Gourmet Roast Beef Pocket (page 77) the next morning to pack for lunch. There's no way you could even go through the drive-thru in the time it takes to wrap up your sandwich. Or what if you made Rigatoni with Meat Sauce (page 100) for dinner, then heated up the leftovers at work? You'd have your co-workers drooling over your lunch, and your hot new figure.

And even if no one else in your household needs to eat better, a little delicious, decadent, healthy food never hurt anyone. And there are plenty of choices that even your picky kids will love. So what are you waiting for? Stop reading and pick up that spatula.

SEE JANE (OR JOHN) RUN

I'd be remiss not to address exercise.

Did you ever notice that when you're not active, you feel sluggish and sometimes even a little less happy than you do after a hard workout or even just a walk outside? For me it's really evident. And the ironic thing is that the more time goes by that I don't work out, the less I feel like doing it. But when I do return, I always think, "Why on earth did I stop?" So what's my trick for jumping back on the treadmill after an absence? I close my eyes and picture myself in a wheelchair in a park with people running and playing. Then I imagine how badly I would long to run if I could never do it again. And when I'm really visualizing that, I always want to be active.

From time to time, I do work out with a trainer. But most of the time, I just try to meet a friend to work out. It's the best way to stay connected to my friends and ensure that workouts happen. If I get to the end of my day and I'm tired, I might convince myself that I don't have the energy. But when I'm looking forward to seeing a friend or he or she is counting on me, I'm far less likely to bail on him or her (or myself!).

Now, don't get me wrong, I'm not a huge stickler. When I travel, I often just don't have a moment at all and I'm okay with that. For instance, one weekend, after flying in the wee hours of the morning, I was facing three straight days of activities from 8 A.M. to 10 P.M. I didn't even take my workout clothes. But when I returned, I made time. The interesting thing is that exercise not only makes me feel better physically, it really sharpens me mentally. So call a friend and schedule that workout. When you're finished you could even cook and eat the most decadent foods ever together.

HOW MUCH WEIGHT WILL YOU LOSE?

The Most Decadent Diet Ever! is tried and true. Every person who has followed this diet has lost weight. And they've all embraced it because it is easy. Many of them could never previously lose weight at all. This book is definitely not about losing ten pounds in ten days. It's about feeling great physically and mentally, today through forever!

After seven years of compulsive, obsessive dieting, in which I gained at least ten to fifteen pounds per year, I started the basis of *The Most Decadent Diet Ever!* I've now maintained a weight loss of more than fifty-five pounds for over sixteen years. I've done more than two hundred interviews and one of the most common questions is "How long did it take you to lose the weight?" Before I answer that question here, I want you to consider a few things: (1) once I lost the weight, I never regained any (except fifteen pounds that I made a conscious decision to regain after actually losing more than seventy pounds; I like that I was blessed with curves that I now actually embrace—they pretty much disappeared when I got down to a size two); (2) I lost more weight

per year than I'd ever previously gained; (3) once I started *The Most Decadent Diet Ever!* my food nightmares stopped (yes, I really had nightmares that had me waking up in a cold sweat thinking I'd eaten an entire cheesecake or warm flourless chocolate cake), and my obsession with food ended; and (4) I started feeling like a normal person for the first time in my life, as I continued to get smaller and smaller and gained more energy. It only took me a few of years of great, scrumptious eating, with constant, noteworthy results, to go from obese to fit. No matter what you have to lose, you will lose and the best part is that you'll be happy, not plagued, through the process.

WHAT DOES *SHE* KNOW?

Reporters often ask me, "Do you think it's hard for people to take advice from you?" Then I quickly tell them that I've lost fifty-five pounds and their tone completely changes. Though, like anyone who's ever had a weight problem, I definitely have my moments, they are extremely few and far between these days, and I know, barring some extreme illness (knock on wood) that I'll never be heavy again. In my early years, I thought I'd never be thin. This is the story of *The Most Decadent Diet Ever!*

It was 1984. I was thirteen years old and I weighed more than 160 pounds. Minutes after Vanessa Williams was crowned Miss America, I locked my bedroom door. Just as in previous years, I put on my bathing suit and my mother's high heels and stood in front of my full-length mirror wondering how on earth *I* was ever going to win that crown.

My grandmother was a beauty pageant winner and even a Miss America contestant back in 1935. Since I inherited her cooking skills, a hint of her singing talents, and her bright smile, I was expected to follow in her footsteps. Every year my mother, my sister, Leslie, and I would watch the pageants, cheering on Miss Pennsylvania. Then, year after year, as the music played and Miss America demonstrated her oh-so-perfect wave with tears streaming down her face, my mom would look at me and say, "That's going to be you some day," with so much love . . . and hope.

So, feeling a bit of pressure, every year I would trudge upstairs to ceremoniously put on my larger-than-last-year's bathing suit to see if there was any way on earth that this was even remotely feasible. And every year as I got fatter and fatter, I saw my mother's Miss America dream slipping away. Then, subconsciously seeking comfort, before I'd even change back to my PJs, I'd grab the peanut brittle that I almost always had stashed under my bed and start munching away.

Now you may be thinking, "Was her mother crazy?" She's not. Not even in the least. She's a Wharton grad and one of those perfectly lovely (and rare) people who see only people's strengths. She set out (emphasis on "set out") to raise the most perfect children on the face of the earth (sorry, Mom). In fact, I was only five when that became blatantly evident to me. My brother and I were going to be the ring bearer and flower girl in my uncle Nick's wedding. So my mom marched us off to Pomeroy's, a local department store, where they offered a "Miss Manners" course that conveniently included lessons on how to walk properly. Though I joke

about it, in retrospect, I'm actually quite grateful for it because it started my media career: by the time I'd finished the course, the department store made me a model and spokesperson for the store.

Though I never managed to compete in the Miss America pageant (trying to buy a bathing suit to go to my school's mandatory pool party was traumatic enough), I somehow thought at sixteen it was a good idea to apply to be a Junior Miss Pageant contestant. Though at the time I weighed at least 180 pounds, people often said, "You have such a pretty face" (granted, the sentiment was always, "What a waste"), and I'd managed to transition from five-year-old model to plus-sized model—with seriously honed walking skills. The Junior Miss Pageant, unlike the Miss America one, was not just a beauty pageant. One girl from each high school competed, and scores were based on beauty, academics, and talent. Since I went to a very small high school and got excellent grades, I actually thought I had a shot. But, alas, Katie Dietrich beat me.

By the time I'd left for college, I'd come to terms with the fact that I'd never actually be a beauty pageant contestant, that I'd never gone to a prom because I was too fat, that I'd never gotten to be a high school cheerleader because I was too fat, and that the closest thing I had to a date by age eighteen was with our plumber's little brother, Jay, who worked at our house from time to time.

After a series of almost-dates with him, which often included him pointing at other girls at the Berkshire Mall with comments like "Don't you wish you looked like her?" he revealed that he'd originally only asked me out as part of a bet, but he later really liked me; that would have been easier to stomach if he hadn't told me that his brother said, "She's frumpy, but cute."

I'd come to terms with the fact that one of the cool guys in my high school class, who didn't give me the time of day, told one of my best friends that I'd be the prettiest girl in the school if I weren't so fat. And I'd come to terms with the fact that Leslie was really thin, really pretty, on the cheerleading squad with straight As, and part of the homecoming court, and had her first boyfriend by the time she was thirteen.

Okay, truth be told, back then I just pretended that I'd come to terms with all of that. I absolutely had not. Needless to say, the pressure was mounting to win my personal battle with the bulge. I was determined, and dieting never worked.

One day I read something that, though I didn't know it at the time, would forever change the course of my life. In retrospect it became sort of my personal "secret" about food: I read that if you cut only 100 calories from your diet per day for an entire year, you'll lose an average of ten pounds in a year. Having dieted for eight years already and never having had even an inkling of success, I found this notion intriguing, especially when you consider that 100 calories is nothing. That's a few bites of a cookie or a tablespoon of creamy salad dressing.

I decided to abandon dieting to try it. And being that I'm a competitive person, I, of course, immediately decided to try to cut 200 or 300 calories from my day—and it worked! For the first time, I was losing weight and I wasn't resentful. I wasn't struggling. I was just skipping a bit of food here or there as I felt like it. And I started using my cooking skills that my grandmother taught me to make simple changes to the foods I loved. I was astounded. And motivated. And within a year, I had lost twenty-five pounds instead of gaining the ten or fifteen I usually gained per year. By the time I graduated from college, I'd lost more than forty pounds.

By the time I was in my early twenties, I had gotten so much pressure to cook for celebrities that I went to culinary school. I immediately fell into owning a catering business specializing in cuisine for a healthy lifestyle. Business was booming and I was a size six. I was teaching celebrities how to cook so they would stay skinny. And people were finding comfort in making my dishes, constantly asking me what I ate, when I ate, how I kept the weight off, and so on. As I taught cooking lessons and did demos at spas around the country, people always asked if I really ate "all of these foods," referring to the foods in my cookbooks, *Fast Food Fix* and *The Biggest Loser Cookbook;* on my show, *Healthy Decadence;* and the recipes in this book. When I said yes, they wanted to know how. *The Most Decadent Diet Ever!* is how.

MY DECADENT PANTRY

I tried to use products throughout this book that are easily found across the country. Many of the products listed here may simply be unfamiliar but are sitting on the shelves at your local grocery store. A few of them may require a trip to a natural foods store, such as Whole Foods. If you're committed to a healthy lifestyle, it's a great idea to peruse the list, picking items that you want to try. Take a trip to a natural foods store and stock your pantry. While you're there, you might even find other healthy treasures.

ancho chile pepper: Found jarred in the spice aisle, it's very similar in heat to cayenne. If your grocery store doesn't carry it, try substituting 1 teaspoon cumin and $^1/_8$ to $^1/_4$ teaspoon cayenne as a second option in Jazzed-Up Jambalaya (page 124).

blue cheese (reduced-fat): Check near the full-fat blue cheese at your favorite grocery store. We often use Treasure Cave brand (treasurecavecheese.com), which is distributed in Wal-Mart, Kroger, and Albertsons stores, among others. If you don't see it, ask the store manager about stocking it or ordering it for you.

Brie (light): Check near other gourmet cheeses. If they don't have it at your local grocery store, try Trader Joe's if that is an option. I use

President brand (presidentcheese.com) and Trader Joe's brand.

burrito seasoning (low-sodium): Look for this near the packets of sauce mixes such as gravy and powdered Alfredo sauce mix. Double-check for the "lower sodium" label, then compare sodium content. Oddly, some brands that are "lower sodium" have as much sodium as other brands that aren't, if not more. Low sodium is 140 milligrams or less per serving. Lower means reduced by at least 25 percent. If you can't find it, you can always use fajita seasoning or taco seasoning.

Cabot's 75% Light Cheddar: Though it's called "light," it's actually more like low-fat, with only 2 $^1/_2$ grams of fat per 1-ounce serving. Look for it with the other block cheeses at your local grocery store or at Trader Joe's. You can use another low-fat variety if you have a favorite. Just be sure it tastes great before you make a whole dish with it.

Cajun seasoning: Look for it in the spice aisle in jars with the other spices or near the Mrs. Dash and other seasonings. Grab the one that is lowest in sodium.

cheese sauce (nacho, reduced-fat, jarred): Frito-Lay makes a really good jarred variety with less sodium than most other brands. Check near the chips or other jarred cheeses at your local grocery store.

chili garlic sauce: Check in the international section of your local grocery store near other

Asian foods such as soy sauce. If you have options, buy the variety with the least sodium.

chipotle peppers in adobo: Look for these in cans in the international section of your local grocery store. They're usually near other Mexican foods such as jarred salsas and canned green chiles.

coconut milk (light): Usually found near Asian foods in the international food aisle of most major grocery stores. If you don't see it, try Whole Foods or another natural foods store, or even Trader Joe's.

couscous (whole-wheat): Look for it near the rice in your local grocery store. If you can't find it, try Whole Foods or another natural foods store.

dried red chile peppers: Usually found in bags in the international foods section of your local grocery store. Some stores stock them else-where, though. If you can't find them, ask. Please note: these peppers are the ones that are about 1 inch long or so.

dried tart cherries: Usually found either in the produce section or with other dried fruit, often near the canned fruits at major grocery stores. If you have trouble finding tart cherries, you can substitute other pitted, dried cherries. Just try to get some that aren't too sweet (check the label for the least amount of added sugar).

edamame (shelled): Check the frozen foods aisle with other frozen vegetables at your grocery store. If you don't see them, try Trader Joe's, Whole Foods, or other natural foods stores.

espresso beans for grinding: Found with other coffees at most grocery stores or your favorite coffee shop—just make sure to buy whole beans. If your espresso has been ground for a while or doesn't have a strong flavor, you may want to double the amount.

feta cheese (reduced-fat): Found at most major grocery stores with traditional packaged feta. Trader Joe's also sells one that's called "light." You'll save even more with the light variety, which also tastes great. Fat-free feta is also an option if you find one you like. Those, however, tend to be hit-and-miss.

grapefruit in lightly sweetened juice: Generally found jarred in the refrigerated case in the produce section. If you can't find it, or want to use unsweetened, you can always peel fresh grapefruit on your own. Work in a bowl and save the juice.

ground chicken breast: If your favorite grocery store doesn't sell it (make sure you're looking for "extra-lean ground chicken" or "ground chicken breast," not just "ground chicken," which may have a lot of fat), go to the meat counter—most butchers will grind boneless, skinless chicken breast for you for no addi-tional charge. Or you can do it yourself by cutting chicken breast into 1-inch cubes and pulsing it in the bowl of a food processor fitted with a chopping blade until it is the same basic consistency as ground meat. Just don't let it become too finely chopped or it will be a purée.

hoisin sauce: Check the international section of your local grocery store near other Asian foods such as soy sauce and sweet-and-sour sauce.

hot sauce (buffalo): I like Frank's RedHot Original Cayenne Pepper Sauce for buffalo wings. It's thicker than some other hot sauces. Look for it near barbecue sauces.

hot sesame oil: Often found next to the toasted sesame oil in the Asian foods section. It may be labeled "hot pepper sesame oil" or "hot chili sesame oil," but don't buy one that just says "hot chili oil." It must say "sesame"! If you can't find it, check a natural foods store such as Whole Foods or an Asian market.

ketchup (low-sodium): Look for it with other ketchups. If you don't see it, check the natural foods aisle, or you can always grab it when you visit a natural foods store such as Whole Foods.

kielbasa or smoked sausage (turkey): Buy the leanest you can find. Check in the deli case with other vacuum-sealed packages of sausage. I use Jennie-O brand turkey kielbasa or turkey smoked sausage (jennieo.com). It has only 3 grams of fat for a 2-ounce serving.

mozzarella (low-fat): Next to the traditional mozzarella; check the label. It should be 2 grams of fat per serving. Lucerne, which is a private label distributed at Safeway, Vons, and Pavilions stores has one.

oat flour (whole-grain): Check the natural foods section near other grains or the baking aisle near other flours at your local grocery store. I often use Bob's Red Mill brand. It's available at bobsredmill.com or at many natural foods stores if not at your local grocery store.

orange peel (dried or dehydrated): Look for it in the spice aisle with other jarred spices and herbs. Natural foods stores such as Whole Foods tend to sell it in bulk if they have a bulk spice section, or you can order it at an online spice store such as Penzey's.

panko bread crumbs (plain or whole-wheat): Often found in the international foods aisle with other Asian foods next to tempura batter. The whole-wheat variety is slighter tougher to find; look for it in the natural foods aisle or natural foods stores such as Whole Foods if it's not with the traditional (white) panko.

queso fresco: Often found in the refrigerated section of major grocery stores not too far from the ricotta and mozzarella cheeses.

red curry paste: Look for it in the international section of your local grocery store near the other Asian foods such as soy sauce.

salt-free Mexican or Southwest seasoning: I often use Mrs. Dash's Southwest Chipotle seasoning, usually found near rubs and seasoning mixes in the spice aisle of most major grocery stores. If you don't see it, ask the manager to order it.

seven-whole-grain pilaf: Oddly enough, this is often in the cereal aisle. If it's not there, check near the rice. Not all grocery stores carry it, so if you can, try Whole Foods or another natural foods store. The one I use is made by Kashi (kashi.com). Other brands also make a pilaf called "whole-grain blend"—this is different. Whole-grain pilaf generally comes in a box and should not have a seasoning packet. Worst-case scenario, substitute short-grain brown rice for the pilaf. The pilaf has three times as much fiber (6 grams for $^1/_2$ cup) and almost three times as much protein, but also has 25 percent more calories.

smoked sausage or kielbasa (turkey): See *kielbasa or smoked sausage (turkey)*.

sugar snap peas: Found in the produce section or at farmers' markets in some parts of the country, but only in season (spring and early summer) in others. If you are unable to find them, substitute Chinese snow peas.

sun-dried tomatoes (not packed in oil): Often in the produce section (not refrigerated) in bags. Trader Joe's and other natural foods stores also sell them.

sweetened condensed milk (fat-free): Found in the baking aisle with other sweetened condensed milk and powdered milk. I use Eagle brand (eaglebrand.com).

taco seasoning (low-sodium): Look near other packets of sauce mixes; double-check for the "lower sodium" label, and then compare the labels. Use burrito or fajita seasoning in a pinch. Or eliminate sodium by using a salt-free Mexican or Southwest seasoning.

toasted sesame oil: Buy one that says "toasted" or "roasted," *not* just "pure sesame oil." Available in the Asian foods section of most major grocery stores. If not, try Whole Foods or another natural foods store.

tortillas (low-fat whole-wheat): Buy a brand that is 96% fat free or more. Also compare and get the one with the least sodium. They're generally found with other tortillas at the ends of aisles in grocery stores or near the deli with other sandwich breads and wraps.

turkey breast (bone-in half): Your local grocery store should carry these, but call ahead if you're unsure. If they don't stock them regularly, talk to your butcher. Most will order them for you at no extra charge.

turkey pepperoni: Most grocery stores carry at least one brand these days. Look with the packaged deli meats or in pouches near the deli counter. If you don't see it, ask.

whole-wheat pastry flour: Check the natural foods section first, but it could also be in the baking aisle. I often use Bob's Red Mill brand (bobsredmill.com). If you can't find it, process whole-wheat flour in the bowl of a food processor fitted with a chopping blade for one to two minutes until very fine.

HELPFUL TOOLS

Though you really don't need much equipment to cook healthy, there are a few essentials that I would definitely recommend.

olive oil sprayer: This absolute must-have is at the top of the list. They cost only about $10. You could use one of the prefilled sprayers you buy at the grocery store in a pinch, but I recommend buying one (check a cooking supply store or a bed-and-bath store) and filling it yourself with your favorite extra virgin olive oil for a couple of reasons. First, the prefilled ones almost always have propellant. Second, I love giving a light mist to foods I bread and bake instead of fry after they come out of the oven. If you use a strong-flavored extra virgin olive oil (another great thing to invest in), the food almost seems fried.

kitchen scale: I've tried to provide equivalents to avoid actually needing a kitchen scale. But it really is good to have one. Though you don't need to weigh and measure everything you're eating all of the time, it's good to do periodic checks to make sure your concept of 4 ounces is actually 4 ounces. I love my digital scale that allows me to zero it out after putting a bowl on it, but any kitchen scale will do. You certainly don't have to spend a lot of money.

nonstick pans: Buy heavy pans with a good nonstick surface. If it's an option, I love Infinite Circulon.

parchment paper: You can always line baking sheets with parchment paper when making unfried items, such as French fries. You'll save a lot of money in the end if you can't (or don't want to) invest in nonstick baking sheets. It's now available at many grocery stores near wax paper. If you don't see it, try a baking store, restaurant supply store, or cooking store.

fine cheese shredder: You'll notice, more often than not, that I call for "finely shredded" low-fat cheese. When you shred lower-fat cheeses finely, they melt better. Plus you'll save calories because you need a lot less to cover the surface area of a food. That way, you'll get some in every bite, adding only a fraction of the amount.

crinkle cutter: Crinkle cutters tend to be oddly inexpensive (between $3.95 and $10 maximum). Check your local cooking store or a bed-and-bath store. Worst-case scenario, do a search online—I found a couple for only $3.95 by typing "crinkle cutter" into a search engine; or you can get a whole garnishing set (to make other foods look pretty) for $9.95.

meat mallet (or rolling pin): When cooking leaner cuts of meat, it's often necessary to take an extra step or two to ensure that the finished dish will be just as tender as the fattier cut. One way is to tenderize, or sometimes flatten, the meat. Buy a mallet with both toothed and flat surfaces—or use a heavy rolling pin in a pinch.

ramekins or small ovenproof glass bowls: I love these because they help with portion control when I can't otherwise help myself. I'm always less likely to dip into seconds than I am to cut a slightly bigger slice of brownie. It's also fun when you're entertaining to serve everyone an individual dessert.

roasting bags (or oven bags): Generally found near zip-top bags and plastic wrap in most major grocery stores.

mini-loaf pans: Lots of grocery stores now sell these near other disposable pans. Or save money by taking a trip to your local restaurant supply store—they always have lots of fun gadgets and equipment that make cooking even more fun. You can also find individual pans at most cooking stores.

KNIFE SKILLS

In case you're new to the kitchen, the following is a quick overview of some of the not-so-obvious cutting you'll need to do to prepare the recipes. Once you follow the directions one time, cutting will become a breeze.

Cutting Meats against the Grain

Meats should always be cut against the grain. When you look at a piece of steak or pork, you can see lines running through it. The longer lines are fibers. When you cut perpendicular to those fibers (not parallel), the knife breaks down the fibers so your teeth have to do a lot less work; the meat is more tender. Also, by cutting thin slices, as opposed to thick ones, you're letting your knife do even more work. Your meat will be as tender as many fattier cuts.

Cutting Carrot Matchsticks

The idea is to cut the carrots so they look like matchsticks—very thin, four-sided strips. Peel the carrot. Then place it on a cutting board and cut a $1/8$-inch-thick lengthwise strip from it so it can lie flat. Place the flat side down, and then continue cutting $1/8$-inch-thick, lengthwise strips until the whole carrot is cut into strips.

Then, stacking a few strips at a time, cut the strips into 1 $1/2$-inch-long pieces. Then cut those pieces lengthwise into $1/8$-inch-thick pieces, stacking them when possible. You should be left with matchsticks.

Cutting Carrot Slivers

Carrot slivers are very similar to carrot matchsticks (see "Cutting Carrot Matchsticks"), though, depending on the recipe, they may be longer (usually up to 2 $1/2$ inches).

Cutting Bell Pepper Slivers

Cut the four faces (sides) from the bell pepper. Discard the core and all of the seeds. Place one face on a cutting board (if your knives aren't super-sharp, it's better to place them facedown). Cut a $1/8$-inch-thick piece from top to bottom. Continue cutting $1/8$-inch-thick pieces. If the pepper was tall, depending on the recipe, you may want to cut the pieces in half crosswise (for a stir-fry, the pieces can be longer; for a chopped salad, shorter is easier to eat).

Cutting Bell Pepper Strips

Bell pepper strips are very similar to bell pepper slivers except that they are thicker and longer. Strips are cut more on preference than slivers or matchsticks. Follow the directions for "Cutting Bell Pepper Slivers," but cut $1/4$-inch to $1/2$-inch pieces.

Cutting Basil Slivers (Chiffonade)

Stack the basil leaves one on top of the other. Then, starting at the end where the stem was attached, roll the leaves tightly, as if you're rolling a blanket in a sleeping bag, yielding a mini-log. Then cut the log crosswise, as thinly as possible, all of the way across. Pull them apart and you'll have basil slivers.

Seeding Cucumbers

Cut the cucumber in half lengthwise. Then use the tip of a spoon to scrape down the center of the cucumber to remove the seeds.

Seeding Tomatoes

Cut the tomato in quarters so that the cuts intersect across the stem end. Use a spoon to scrape the seeds and the insides from the tomato, leaving the thick outer portion (the meat) intact. Discard the seeds and insides. Cut the cores from the quarters and discard them. You're now ready to cut the meat into whatever size pieces the recipe requires.

GET GRILLING

I love grilling. It's a great way to add flavor to food without adding fat and calories. Throughout this book, I sometimes give instructions to "Preheat a grill to high." This can be whatever kind of grill you have (or one that you can use based on the weather). I use a gas grill because I prefer it over indoor grilling and I live in a condo, so I couldn't have a charcoal grill even if I wanted to have one. If you, like my dad, enjoy the experience of getting the coals just so, lighting them, and feeding a fire, that's perfect. But here's a little guidance when cooking meats and chicken no matter which grill you have:

gas grill: When cooking meats like steak or a pork roast, always set the grill to high and leave it on high. You want to cook the meat for a short time over high heat. With chicken, preheat the grill to high, and then as soon as you put the chicken on, turn the heat to medium. Boneless, skinless chicken breasts (the only kind I use throughout the book) have virtually no fat content, so cooking them through on high heat could dry them out. Starting on high but turning the heat down will sear the outside without charring it as the chicken cooks through.

charcoal grill: With a charcoal grill, light the coals and let the flame get going. When the grill is hot, add fattier meats like steak right over the direct flame. Place skinless chicken breasts and other super-lean meats on the outer edges of the grill rack, so as not to dry them out.

indoor grill: If you have an indoor grill that uses coals or some other means to add grilled flavor, that's ideal. A tabletop grill is okay as a second option. The kind with a flat surface where you have to flip the meat is best; the ones that sandwich the meat tend to steam it, making it less juicy, and the outsides never get that browned crust that tastes so good.

If you're using a flat indoor grill, preheat it to high. Place the meat on the grill and sear it about one to two minutes per side. Then continue cooking until it is done throughout—if it starts getting too dark on the outside, simply turn the heat to medium to allow the meat to continue cooking until it reaches the desired doneness or, in the case of chicken, until it is no longer pink inside.

breakfasts

WE'VE HEARD IT OVER AND OVER: breakfast is the most important meal of the day. As much as I resisted the notion for years, I truly believe it is. When I was overweight, I was never hungry in the morning (probably because I ate too much at night).

Some days I "made it" until afternoon without eating, and I thought that was a good thing. But when I'd cut my calories down so that I should have been losing weight and wasn't, I went to a nutritionist. She was sure I'd lose weight if I ate early in the day. My big fear was that if I started eating earlier, I'd eat way too much, since I've always been a late-afternoon and early-evening eater. Finally, after much pressure, she convinced me that if I woke up and had just two bites of a banana, it couldn't possibly kill my caloric intake for the day and it would help kick-start my metabolism early.

She was right. I started with that and then added a small snack in the morning—that's all that felt safe at the time—and I started losing quicker. Now I eat five meals a day that are spread out throughout the day when I'm not in my kitchen. When I am cooking, I eat a few bites here and there all day. The latter is not ideal, but it's the one really challenging part of my work. If I can endure that and maintain my weight loss, you can do it too!

1 2 Chocolate Chip Pancakes
1 2 Orange Raspberry Pancakes
3 Sausage Biscuit Sandwich
2 Quick Canadian Bacon and Egg Breakfast Sandwich
2 Fried Egg in Olive Bread
3 Five-Minute Supreme Breakfast Nachos
2 French Toast with Sautéed Banana
2 Vanilla, Chocolate, and Strawberry Breakfast Sundae
1 2 Bacon Swiss Omelet
2 Devin's Eggs
2 Western Skinny Scramble
2 Scrambled Eggs with Sautéed Shrimp
3 Bacon and Egg Breakfast Quesadilla
1 Breakfast Sausage Links
1 2 Potatoes O'Brien
3 Chocolate Peanut Butter Breakfast "Pudding"
2 Lemon-Blueberry Oatmeal
1 Banana-Coconut Mini-Muffins
2 Sinless Yet Sinful Sticky Buns
1 2 Banana Colada Smoothie
2 Cinnamon Apple Yogurt Parfait

CHOCOLATE CHIP PANCAKES

Aaah, chocolate for breakfast, what could be more heavenly? One of my downfalls has always been warm chocolate chip cookies. I just love those slightly melty chips! This recipe is my solution to that chocolate chip craving, guilt free. These pancakes are chock-full of chocolate chips, so I actually prefer them without butter. But if you like a more buttery taste with just a hint of chips, use only 1 tablespoon of chips and spread 1 teaspoon of light butter over the top of each pancake. You'll add 17 calories and 2 grams of fat per teaspoon. You'll also notice that the recipe calls for very little syrup. Each teaspoon has 17 calories and 0 grams of fat. If you love syrup and want to add more, you can. Just try the pancakes first and then add only as little syrup as you possibly can to feel that you're eating a truly decadent meal. Being a true chocolate lover, I prefer them exactly as is.

If you're harried like most, you can double or triple this recipe with great success. The batter will keep in your refrigerator for up to three days, which will save time in the mornings.

1 large egg white, lightly beaten
$^1/_2$ cup low-fat buttermilk
$^1/_2$ cup whole-grain oat flour (see page 17)

$^1/_2$ teaspoon baking soda
$^1/_4$ teaspoon vanilla extract
$^1/_8$ teaspoon salt
2 tablespoons mini chocolate chips
Butter-flavored cooking spray
4 teaspoons pure maple syrup, divided

Preheat the oven to 200°F.

Whisk the egg white, buttermilk, flour, baking soda, vanilla, and salt in a small mixing bowl. Stir in $1^1/_2$ tablespoons water until well incorporated. Then stir in the chocolate chips and let stand for 10 minutes.

Preheat a large nonstick skillet over medium-high heat. When a spritz of water causes the skillet to sizzle, working in batches and respraying between each batch, mist the skillet with spray and pour $^1/_4$ cup of batter per pancake onto the skillet. Cook until there are bubbles on the top and the bottom is golden brown, about 2 minutes. Flip each pancake and cook until lightly golden brown on the bottom, about another 2 minutes. Transfer the finished pancakes to an ovenproof plate, cover with foil, and keep them warm in the oven until they are all cooked. Serve immediately with 1 teaspoon maple syrup per pancake.

Can be made in 30 minutes or less / No more than 20 minutes hands-on prep time

MAKES 4 PANCAKES; 2 SERVINGS OR 4 PORTIONS

Each 1-Decadent-Disk portion (1 pancake) has: 105 calories, 4 g protein, 16 g carbohydrates, 3 g fat, 1 g saturated fat, 2 mg cholesterol, 1 g fiber, 272 mg sodium

Each 2-Decadent-Disk serving (2 pancakes) has: 209 calories, 8 g protein, 31 g carbohydrates, 6 g fat, 3 g saturated fat, 5 mg cholesterol, 3 g fiber, 544 mg sodium

You save: 218 calories, 17 g fat, 3 g saturated fat

Traditional serving: 427 calories, 9 g protein, 51 g carbohydrates, 23 g fat, 6 g saturated fat, 117 mg cholesterol, fiber N/A, 470 mg sodium

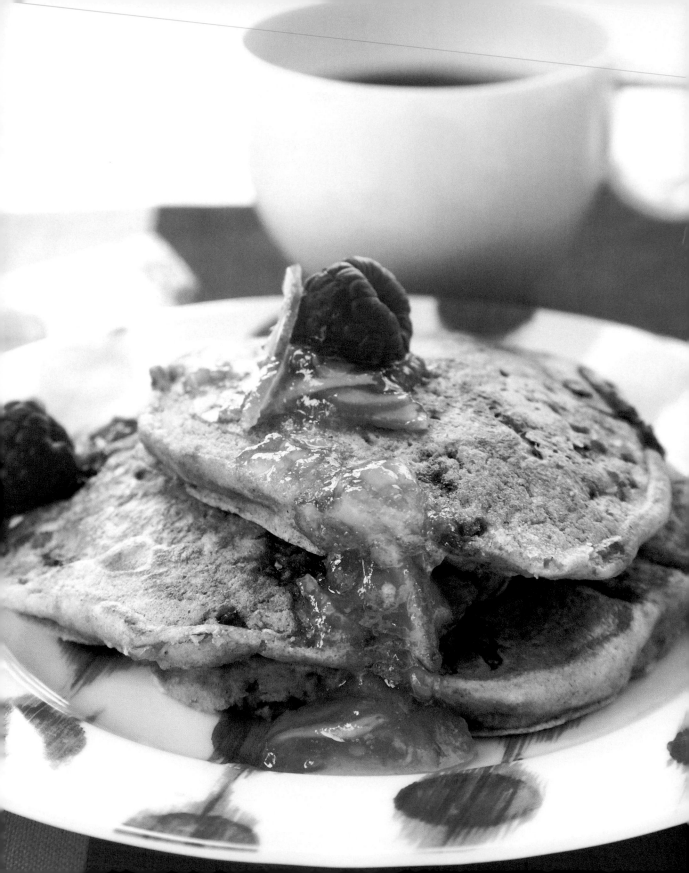

ORANGE RASPBERRY PANCAKES

1 **2**

I'm single ... and I am the queen of befriending women. Though I'd love to meet a great guy, no matter where I go or what I do, I walk away with a new female friend. I even tried speed dating; I didn't hit it off with any of the men, but the woman who ran it, Christina, quickly became one of my best friends.

Christina loves to cook and entertain. One weekend, she had a brunch and made the most amazing orange raspberry pancakes. I only had a piece of a pancake because they were a bit fattening for me, but I kept thinking about them, so I recreated them using whole grain oat flour and less fat. One of these days I may end up with a husband; for now, at least I have the best girlfriends in the world!

$^1/_2$ cup frozen raspberries
1 teaspoon sugar
1 large egg white, lightly beaten
$^1/_2$ cup low-fat buttermilk
$^1/_2$ cup whole-grain oat flour (see page 17)
$^1/_2$ teaspoon baking soda
$^1/_2$ teaspoon orange extract
$^1/_4$ teaspoon vanilla extract
$^1/_8$ teaspoon salt
$^1/_4$ teaspoon dried orange peel
Butter-flavored cooking spray

4 teaspoons pure maple syrup or 2 tablespoons 100% fruit orange marmalade
Fresh raspberries, optional

Preheat the oven to 200°F.

Put the frozen raspberries in a sieve and allow them to defrost in the sink, or microwave on low for about 30 seconds until defrosted, and then drain them. Coarsely chop the raspberries and transfer them to a small bowl. Add the sugar and stir until well combined.

Whisk the egg white, buttermilk, flour, baking soda, orange extract, vanilla, salt, and orange peel in a small mixing bowl. Stir in the raspberries and let stand for 10 minutes.

Preheat a large nonstick skillet over medium-high heat. When a spritz of water causes the skillet to sizzle, working in batches and respraying between each batch, mist the skillet with spray and pour $^1/_4$ cup of batter per pancake onto the skillet. Cook until there are bubbles on the top and the bottom is golden brown, about 2 minutes. Flip each pancake and cook until lightly golden brown on the bottom, about another 2 minutes. Transfer the finished pancakes to an ovenproof plate, cover with foil, and keep them warm in the oven until they are all cooked. Serve immediately with 1 teaspoon maple syrup or $1^1/_2$ teaspoons marmalade per pancake. Garnish with raspberries, if desired.

Can be made in 30 minutes or less / No more than 20 minutes hands-on prep time

MAKES 4 PANCAKES; 2 SERVINGS OR 4 PORTIONS

1 Each 1-Decadent-Disk portion (1 pancake) has: 98 calories, 4 g protein, 18 g carbohydrates, 2 g fat, trace saturated fat, 2 mg cholesterol, 2 g fiber, 278 mg sodium

2 Each 2-Decadent-Disk serving (2 pancakes) has: 197 calories, 7 g protein, 35 g carbohydrates, 3 g fat, <1 g saturated fat, 4 mg cholesterol, 4 g fiber, 557 mg sodium

SAUSAGE BISCUIT SANDWICH

3

If you were to tell me that I could eat any breakfast without consequence any time, I'd likely choose a sausage biscuit sandwich with egg that was dripping with cheese. There's something about that combo in the morning that I just love. Here's one that's sensible. But when I say "sensible," don't mistake that for small. This sandwich, when assembled, weighs a full 8 ounces. Though it has much less fat, many fewer calories, and even significantly less sodium than any you could grab at a drive-thru, it's even larger than the large size at most. Plus it adds plenty of protein.

In the recipe, I instruct you to make the sausage mixture from the Breakfast Sausage Links, but omit $^1/_4$ teaspoon of salt when doing so. Eaten on its own, this sausage needs at least that much salt to compare to ones you'd buy. But in this sandwich, the biscuit is a bit salty so you don't need the extra salt.

If you love this sandwich as much as I do and need a quick, before-work option, simply freeze the baked biscuits and freeze the patties separately in a single layer or stacked between sheets of wax paper in an airtight container. The patties will "fry" up quickly and the biscuits can be wrapped completely in foil and reheated in a 400° oven while you shower, do your makeup, or shave. You'll need only five minutes hands-on in the morning, which is less time than it would take to sit in the line at the drive-thru.

1 recipe **Better Buttermilk Biscuits dough**
    (page 225)
$^3/_4$ **recipe Breakfast Sausage Links mixture,**
    unshaped (page 44)
Olive oil spray
5 large egg whites

MAKES 5 SANDWICHES; 5 SERVINGS

3 Each 3-Decadent-Disk serving (1 sandwich) has: 306 calories, 26 g protein, 35 g carbohydrates, 8 g fat, 3 g saturated fat, 66 mg cholesterol, 2 g fiber, 767 mg sodium

You save: 194 calories, 23 g fat, 7 g saturated fat

Traditional serving: 500 calories, 10 g protein, 36 g carbohydrates, 31 g fat, 10 g saturated fat, 250 mg cholesterol, 1 g fiber, 1,080 mg sodium

Make the dough for the Better Buttermilk Biscuits. Continue to follow the directions but instead of forming 6 biscuits, use a knife or pastry cutter to cut the rectangle of dough into 5 equal pieces. With your hands, shape each piece into a $3^1/_2$-inch-diameter biscuit to make 5 biscuits. Bake for 15 to 17 minutes instead of 13 to 15.

Meanwhile, prepare the Breakfast Sausage Links mixture, omitting $^1/_4$ teaspoon of the salt (use only $^1/_4$ teaspoon total). Divide the mixture into 5 equal parts, and then shape each into a ball. Flatten one of the balls into a 4-inch-diameter patty on a sheet of wax paper. Repeat with the remaining balls, forming each into a patty.

Preheat a large nonstick skillet over high heat. Lightly mist it with spray and add the patties, side by side. Cook for 1 to 2 minutes per side, until lightly browned on the outside. Turn the heat to medium and cook for another 1 to 3 minutes, until just barely pink inside.

Transfer the patties to a plate and cover to keep warm.

Respray the skillet and return the heat to medium-high. Add the egg whites, one at a time, working in batches if necessary, to "fry" them, making sure they do not run together (pour into a $3^1/_2$-inch-diameter cookie cutter lightly misted with spray or a hollowed-out tuna can, if desired). When the bottoms are set, after about 1 minute, flip and continue cooking until set throughout.

Cut each biscuit in half and place the bottom half, inside faceup, on a plate. Add one egg to each, followed by one sausage patty. Place the biscuit tops atop each. Serve immediately.

Note how much protein is in the *Most Decadent Diet Ever!* version compared to the traditional. Though both have virtually the same amount of carbohydrates, my version uses a much bigger sausage patty for added protein with way less fat and calories.

QUICK CANADIAN BACON AND EGG BREAKFAST SANDWICH

2

It's really important to get lots of fiber in your diet. Fiber helps you fill up without filling out. Obviously, eating lots of veggies is one way to get your needed fiber intake, but you can also get fiber from fruits, whole grains, and some great new products found on the shelves at grocery stores all over the country. One of the products I love best are light English muffins, which often contain lots of fiber. I also love high-fiber tortillas and fiber-enriched pasta. Recently, I've found a lot of granola-type bars that pack in the fiber. Those are great to curb hunger, especially when you just don't have time to cook and need a little pick-me-up in the middle of the day or before or after a workout.

I love this sandwich on the light English muffin. If you can't find them, or just prefer to swap out the light one for a whole-grain one, you can do that. But then you should skip the cheese to keep it to a 200-calorie sandwich.

Olive oil spray
1 large egg white
1 light English muffin
1 slice ($^3/_4$ ounce) Canadian bacon, heated if desired
1 slice ($^3/_4$ ounce) 2% milk American cheese

Lightly mist a $3^1/_2$- or 4-inch-diameter ramekin or microwave-safe bowl with spray. Put the egg white in the ramekin.

Toast the English muffin in a toaster or under the broiler.

Microwave the egg white on low in 15-second intervals until it is no longer runny. Then assemble the sandwich by placing the bottom half of the English muffin, inside faceup, on a plate. Top it with the bacon, the egg, the cheese, and the top half of the muffin. If desired, wrap the sandwich in wax paper and microwave on low for 15 to 30 seconds to melt the cheese. Serve immediately.

Can be made in 30 minutes or less / No more than 20 minutes hands-on prep time

MAKES 1 SANDWICH; 1 SERVING

 Each 2-Decadent-Disk serving (1 sandwich) has: 208 calories, 21 g protein, 26 g carbohydrates, 6 g fat, 2 g saturated fat, 22 mg cholesterol, 8 g fiber, 757 mg sodium
You save: 152 calories, 10 g fat, 4 g saturated fat
Traditional serving: 360 calories, 17 g protein, 36 g carbohydrates, 16 g fat, 6 g saturated fat, 200 mg cholesterol, 1 g fiber, 1,300 mg sodium

FRIED EGG IN OLIVE BREAD

2

My favorite bread has always been olive bread. Truth be told, if olives didn't have so much salt coupled with lots of fat (granted, it is "good fat," but still), I would have included at least another handful of recipes where they were prominent. I just love them. So this recipe is a bit of an homage to them. I've never actually seen toad-in-the-hole served in olive bread, but have always thought it should be.

If you can't find a loaf of olive bread that is the exact dimension of the one listed, don't worry. The gist here is to consume 2 ounces of bread and 2 egg whites.

Two 1-ounce oval slices olive bread (each about
$^1/_2$ inch thick, $2^1/_4$ X $4^1/_4$ inches)
1 teaspoon light butter, divided
2 large egg whites
Olive oil spray
Salt and pepper

Butter one side of a slice of bread with $^1/_2$ teaspoon butter. Use a cookie cutter or a knife to carefully cut out an oval from the center of the bread, about 3 inches by 1 inch. Remove the oval piece from the center and set aside. Repeat with the second slice of bread and the remaining butter.

Crack each egg white into a separate small bowl.

Preheat a medium nonstick skillet over medium-high heat until it is hot enough for a spritz of water to sizzle on it. Mist the skillet with spray and quickly lay the bread slices side by side, buttered side up, in the skillet. Next, slowly pour 1 egg white into the center of each slice of bread, being careful not to let the egg run out of the hole. Season each egg white with salt and pepper to taste.

Lay the reserved oval cutouts, buttered side up, next to the bread slices in the pan.

When the egg whites begin to set around the edges of the holes, flip the bread and reduce the heat to medium. Season the other sides with salt and pepper to taste and cook until the egg whites are completely set and the bread slices are toasted, 2 to 4 minutes.

Meanwhile, flip the oval cutouts and cook until toasted, 2 to 3 minutes. Serve immediately.

Can be made in 30 minutes or less / No more than 20 minutes hands-on prep time

MAKES 1 SERVING

2 Each 2-Decadent-Disk serving (2 slices) has: 204 calories, 11 g protein, 28 g carbohydrates, 5 g fat, 1 g saturated fat, 5 mg cholesterol, 0 g fiber, 553 mg sodium

FIVE-MINUTE SUPREME BREAKFAST NACHOS

3

Though I'm definitely a "relationship girl," one of the few things I love about being single is that it almost forces me to try new restaurants. When a date asks me where I want to eat, I always tell him to pick his favorite spot. That way, even if I don't hit it off with him, I can scour the menu to find a unique dish that might be fun to transform.

These nachos are the result of a leisurely Sunday morning date by the beach. We met at a little café and he ordered the breakfast nachos. I was excited about his choice because I knew I wouldn't eat traditional nacho chips since they're deep-fried, but I wanted to see the dish.

It was as appealing as I thought it would be. And now I can eat it too, since my version is much healthier. It's likely you'll like it as much as I do.

1 ounce lightly salted, baked tortilla chips (about 14 chips)

2 tablespoons salsa verde

1¹/₂ tablespoons red taco sauce

2 tablespoons plus 2 teaspoons jarred reduced-fat zesty cheese sauce

Olive oil spray

4 large egg whites

Salt and pepper

³/₄ cup coarsely chopped tomatoes

Spread half of the tortilla chips evenly in the bottom of a medium shallow bowl.

Combine the salsa and taco sauce in a small microwave-safe bowl.

Pour the cheese sauce into a second small microwave-safe bowl.

Mist a third small microwave-safe bowl with spray. Add the egg whites and season with salt and pepper to taste. Microwave all three bowls on low for 30 seconds. Remove the salsa mixture and cheese sauce when they are hot (be careful not to overcook the cheese—it won't melt). Continue microwaving the eggs in 30-second intervals until they are just a bit runny on top. Then stir with a fork, breaking them apart into large pieces. By the time you "scramble" and stir them, the residual heat should have cooked away the runniness. If they are still undercooked, microwave them on low in 10-second intervals until just done.

Spread half of the scrambled eggs over the chips. Then drizzle half of the cheese sauce over that. Spread the second layer of tortillas on top, followed by the remaining eggs and the remaining cheese sauce. Spoon the salsa mixture evenly over the center. Sprinkle the tomatoes evenly over the top of the salsa mixture. Serve immediately.

Can be made in 30 minutes or less / No more than 20 minutes hands-on prep time

MAKES 1 SERVING

3 Each 3-Decadent-Disk serving has: 292 calories, 20 g protein, 38 g carbohydrates, 5 g fat, 2 g saturated fat, 5 mg cholesterol, 4 g fiber, 812 mg sodium

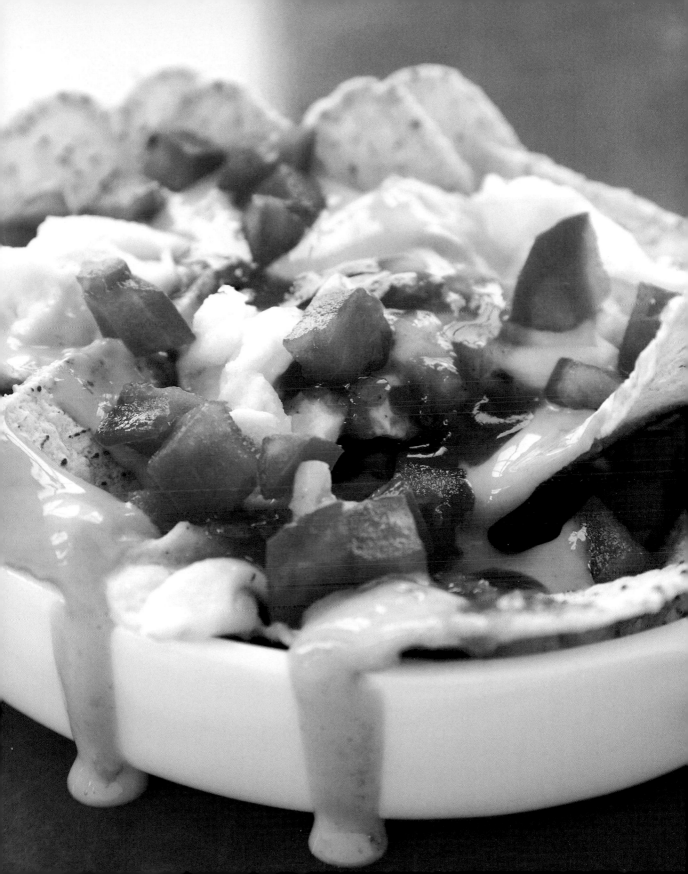

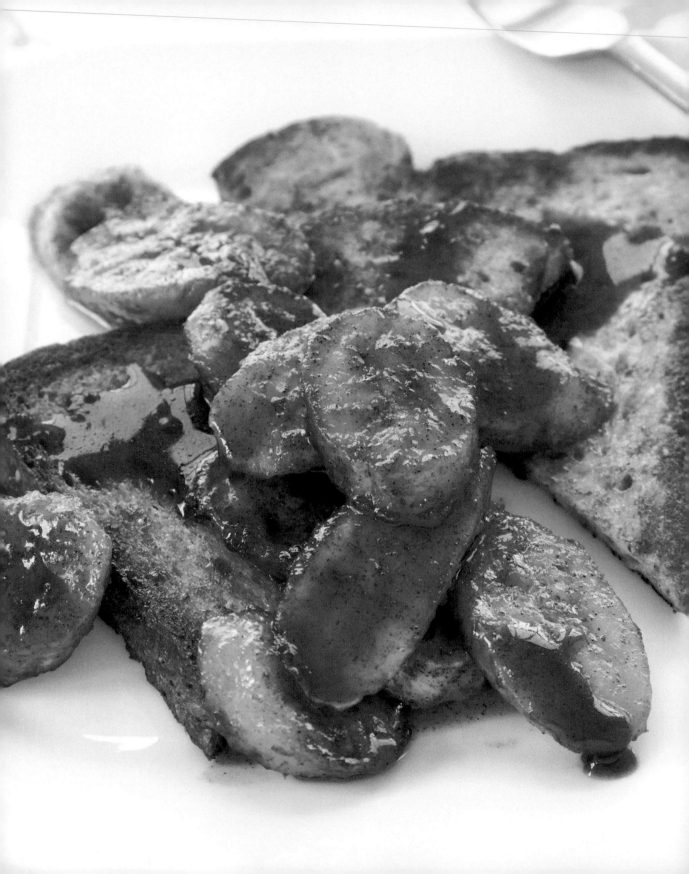

FRENCH TOAST WITH SAUTÉED BANANA

2

Over the past year or so, I've gotten slightly addicted to cooking fruit—it's really amazing how heat can bring out the natural sugars. It all started when my friend Rasha, who was one of the contestants on the "Engaged Couples" special episode of *The Biggest Loser*, sent me a recipe for baked grapefruit that I included in *The Biggest Loser Cookbook*. All she did was bake the grapefruit with a little bit of cinnamon and sweetener on the top, and it was suddenly transformed from the same ol', same ol' into such a treat. That inspired me to roast pineapple (see Roasted Pineapple à la Mode, page 221), which is also exceptionally satisfying. And now, here's another dish with warmed fruit. This one definitely helps start your day on an indulgent note, while helping your quest to get much-needed fruits and veggies in your diet.

For the banana
1 medium firm banana
1 tablespoon sugar
$1/2$ teaspoon fresh lemon juice
$1/4$ teaspoon ground cinnamon
2 teaspoons light butter

Peel the banana and cut it on a diagonal, creating $1/4$-inch-thick slices. Transfer the slices to a medium bowl and add the sugar, lemon juice, and cinnamon. Toss to coat evenly.

Place a small nonstick skillet over medium-high heat. Put in the butter. When it bubbles ever so slightly, add the banana slices. Cook, stirring frequently, until tender and slightly caramel-ized, 2 to 4 minutes. Remove from the heat and cover to keep it warm.

For the French toast
$1/4$ cup fat-free milk
2 tablespoons egg substitute
$1^{1}/2$ teaspoons sugar
$1/4$ teaspoon ground cinnamon
1 teaspoon light butter
2 slices whole-wheat bread

Mix the milk, egg substitute, sugar, and cinnamon in a large shallow bowl.

Preheat a large nonstick skillet over medium-high heat. Put in the butter.

Soak one slice of bread in the egg mixture until just soft, turning once. Let any excess egg mixture drip off and transfer the bread to one side of the skillet. Repeat with the second slice of bread, placing it next to the first slice in the skillet. Cook for 1 to 3 minutes per side, until golden brown on both sides. Transfer each piece to a plate and top each with half of the banana mixture. Serve immediately.

Can be made in 30 minutes or less / No more than 20 minutes hands-on prep time

MAKES 2 SERVINGS

2 Each 2-Decadent-Disk serving (1 slice) has: 202 calories, 6 g protein, 40 g carbohydrates, 4 g fat, 2 g saturated fat, 8 mg cholesterol, 4 g fiber, 244 mg sodium

You save: 156 calories, 9 g fat, 4 g saturated fat

Traditional serving: 358 calories, 10 g protein, 49 g carbohydrates, 13 g fat, 6 g saturated fat, 127 mg cholesterol, 3 g fiber, 566 mg sodium

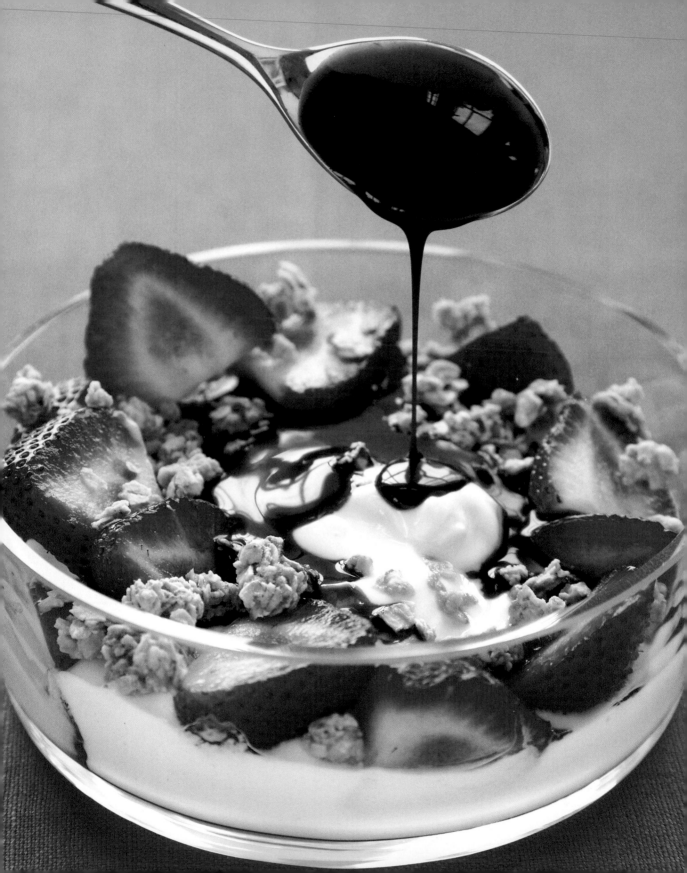

VANILLA, CHOCOLATE, AND STRAWBERRY BREAKFAST SUNDAE

2

I was recently in Chicago for a culinary conference. I went to breakfast with one of the publicists from my TV show, *Healthy Decadence*. Though I normally read every word on every menu presented to me (a definite foodie quirk!), I was a bit distracted preparing for a TV appearance. When the waiter came along and asked Anna what she'd like, she said, "The Vanilla Strawberry Breakfast Sundae." Intrigued (and surprised I had missed it), I couldn't wait to see her plate. It was quite disappointing really, but it set my wheels turning. It sounded (*sounded*, in this case, being the operative word) like something I'd want to eat. So being true to my near obsession with chocolate, I tweaked it, and then added some chocolate. My friends and I have since eaten this three-minute-throw-together breakfast over and over.

If you prefer not to eat artificially sweetened yogurt, you don't have to. Substituting a low-fat (I haven't seen it in fat free), naturally sweetened one adds 70 to 80 calories and 2 grams of fat to this dish.

^{2}/$_3$ cup fat-free, artificially sweetened vanilla yogurt
3 tablespoons low-fat granola without raisins
^{1}/$_4$ cup sliced strawberries
1^1/$_2$ teaspoons chocolate syrup

Spoon the yogurt into a small, deep bowl (about 5 inches in diameter). Sprinkle the granola evenly over the yogurt. Top the granola with the strawberries, and then drizzle evenly with the chocolate syrup. Serve immediately.

Can be made in 30 minutes or less / No more than 20 minutes hands-on prep time

MAKES 1 SUNDAE; 1 SERVING

2 Each 2-Decadent-Disk serving (1 sundae) has: 197 calories, 7 g protein, 40 g carbohydrates, 1 g fat, trace saturated fat, 3 mg cholesterol, 2 g fiber, 144 mg sodium

BACON SWISS OMELET

⚡1⚡ ⚡2⚡

Let's face it, Americans love bacon. We all know it: everything tastes better with bacon. And most of us indulge. We eat it for breakfast, top casseroles with it, and even wrap our veggies in it. Though I love it, I had stopped eating bacon entirely when I started losing weight. I must have gone a few years without having even a bite. Then I realized that center-cut bacon (it's real pork bacon and can be found in most major grocery stores with the rest of the bacon) has about 40 percent less fat than traditional bacon. In fact, it has less fat than even some brands and varieties of turkey bacon. These days I still eat it sparingly, because of its high salt content, but I do eat it. This omelet has quickly become one of my favorites. Not only does it taste great, it's a substantial omelet that, coupled with a piece of fruit or a cup of On-the-Terrace Fruit Salad (page 222), keeps me full for hours.

2 slices center-cut bacon, chopped

^{1}/4 cup chopped sweet onion

4 large egg whites

1^1/2 teaspoons chopped fresh parsley

Salt and pepper

Olive oil spray

1 ounce (about ^{1}/3 cup) finely shredded light Swiss cheese

Place a small nonstick skillet over medium-high heat. Put in the bacon and cook, stirring occasionally, until very crisp, 5 to 7 minutes. Transfer to a small bowl lined with a paper towel, and cover to keep warm. Reduce the heat to medium, and then return the skillet to the heat and add the onion (a little bacon grease should remain). Cook until tender, about 5 minutes. Add the onion to the bacon and remove the skillet from the heat.

Combine the egg whites with the parsley in a small bowl. Season with salt and pepper to taste. Whisk until the egg whites bubble lightly.

Place a medium nonstick skillet over medium heat. When the skillet is warm, lightly mist it with spray and pour the egg mixture into the skillet. Cook, lifting the edges with a spatula as they start to set. Tip the skillet, allowing the uncooked egg to run underneath, and cook until almost set, 4 to 6 minutes. Flip the omelet. Sprinkle the bacon mixture and cheese evenly over half of the egg. Fold the bare half over the filled half and continue cooking the omelet until the cheese is just melted. Transfer to a plate or cut in half and divide between 2 plates and serve immediately.

Can be made in 30 minutes or less / No more than 20 minutes hands-on prep time

MAKES 1 OMELET; 1 SERVING OR 2 PORTIONS

⚡1⚡ Each 1-Decadent-Disk portion (^{1}/2 omelet) has: 103 calories, 14 g protein, 2 g carbohydrates, 4 g fat, 2 g saturated fat, 12 mg cholesterol, trace fiber, 302 mg sodium

⚡2⚡ Each 2-Decadent-Disk serving (1 omelet) has: 206 calories, 28 g protein, 5 g carbohydrates, 8 g fat, 4 g saturated fat, 24 mg cholesterol, <1 g fiber, 603 mg sodium

You save: 269 calories, 30 g fat, 12 g saturated fat

Traditional serving: 475 calories, 27 g protein, 5 g carbohydrates, 38 g fat, 16 g saturated fat, 484 mg cholesterol, 0 g fiber, 554 mg sodium

DEVIN'S EGGS

Every time we had overnight guests when I was growing up, my mom served a dish called Jenny's Eggs. It was from a recipe she had gotten from my aunt JoAnne for what was basically a crustless quiche. It had a pound of cheese, at least a stick or two of butter, tons of whole eggs, and plenty of ham. It was delicious, but virtually lethal. My mom particularly loved to serve it to company because you prepare the dish the night before, then look like the perfect hostess in the morning when your guests wake up to the smell of the delicious casserole and walk into a spotless kitchen. I, of course, loved the concept, because I also entertain often. But you'd never catch me eating those ingredients these days. So here is my version, aptly renamed Devin's Eggs.

If you can't find lean ham steak at your grocery store, go to the deli counter and ask them to slice a $1/4$-inch-thick slice of the leanest ham they have. Also try for a low-sodium variety if they have it. Then simply chop $5^1/2$ ounces of that into cubes.

Olive oil spray

$1^1/2$ cups finely chopped red or yellow onion

1 cup finely chopped red or green bell pepper, or a combination

6 slices whole-wheat bread, cubed (from a light, fluffy loaf, not a dense one; about 70 calories per slice)

5 ounces (about 2 cups) finely shredded Cabot's 75% Light Cheddar cheese, or your favorite low-fat Cheddar

$5^1/2$ ounces (about $1^1/4$ cups) 98% lean ham steak, cut into $1/4$-inch cubes

$2^1/2$ cups egg substitute

$1/4$ cup fat-free milk

2 teaspoons dry mustard

$1/2$ teaspoon black pepper

$1/8$ teaspoon salt

(continued)

No more than 20 minutes hands-on prep time

MAKES 1 CASSEROLE; 6 SERVINGS

Each 2-Decadent-Disk serving ($1/6$ casserole) has: 209 calories, 23 g protein, 22 g carbohydrates, 4 g fat, 1 g saturated fat, 18 mg cholesterol, 3 g fiber, 740 mg sodium

You save: 247 calories, 23 g fat, 14 g saturated fat

Traditional version: 456 calories, 22 g protein, 30 g carbohydrates, 27 g fat, 15 g saturated fat, 178 mg cholesterol, fiber N/A, 824 mg sodium

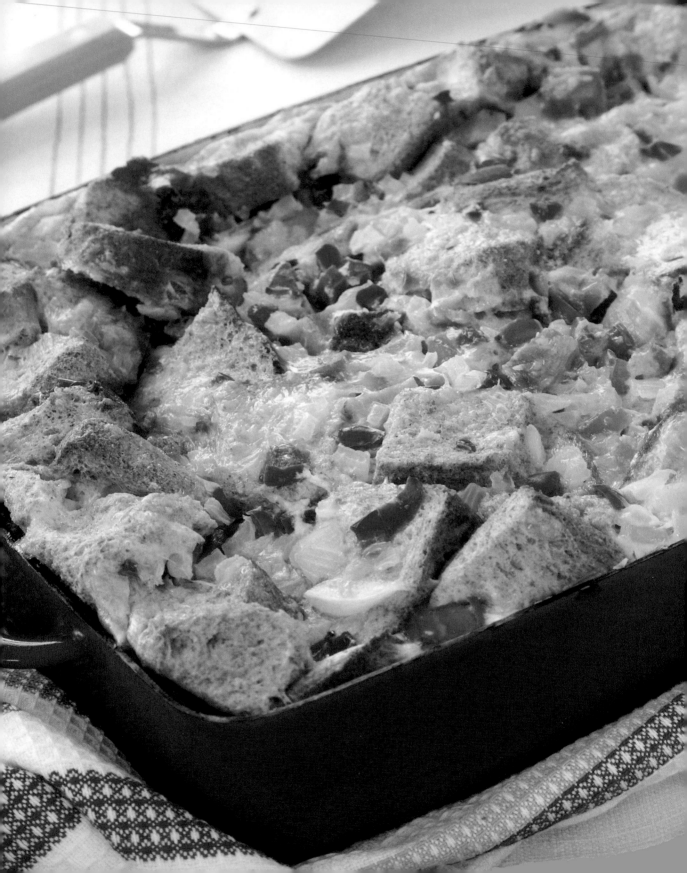

Lightly mist a medium nonstick skillet with spray and place it over medium heat. Put in the onion and bell pepper. Cook until the veggies are tender and the excess liquid has evaporated, about 5 minutes.

Meanwhile, lightly mist an 11 X 7-inch ovenproof glass or ceramic baking dish with spray. Spread half of the bread evenly in the dish to form a layer. Then evenly layer half of the cheese, followed by half of the onion mixture, then half of the ham. Repeat with the remaining ingredients, making sure that they are evenly distributed all the way to the edges of the dish and not mounded in the center. Set aside.

Combine the egg substitute, milk, mustard, black pepper, and salt in a large measuring cup or medium bowl. Whisk until thoroughly mixed. Pour the egg mixture over the bread, cheese, veggies, and ham. Use a fork to very gently press the ingredients into the liquid without mashing them. Cover with plastic wrap and refrigerate overnight.

Preheat the oven to 350°F.

Remove the plastic wrap and bake for 40 to 45 minutes, until the egg is set in the center. Remove from the oven and let stand for 5 to 10 minutes. Cut the casserole into 6 pieces and serve immediately.

WESTERN SKINNY SCRAMBLE

My friend Leigh told me years ago that her favorite breakfast was from her gym. She described the clerk behind the food bar making scrambled egg whites in the microwave. It sounded perfectly awful to me. But she insisted that it truly was the base of the best scrambled egg whites she'd ever had. As a chef, I rarely use a microwave to cook anything. Sure, I do a bit of reheating here and there. But intrigued, I decided to give it a try. Not only were the eggs quite tasty, they were even better than most egg whites I'd made in pans. Add these few ingredients and you're set to have a satisfying meal in moments, gym-style.

Olive oil spray
4 large egg whites
1 ounce (about ¹/₄ cup) ¹/₄-inch Canadian bacon cubes
¹/₃ cup chopped onion
¹/₃ cup chopped green bell pepper
1 ounce (about ¹/₂ cup) finely shredded Cabot's 75% Light Cheddar cheese, or your favorite low-fat Cheddar
Salt and pepper

Lightly mist a medium microwave-safe bowl with spray. Put in the egg whites.

Preheat a small nonstick skillet over medium-high heat. Lightly mist it with spray. Place the bacon, onion, and bell pepper in the skillet. Cook, stirring with a wooden spoon, until the onion and bell pepper are tender, but not browned, 6 to 8 minutes.

Meanwhile, microwave the egg whites on low for 30 seconds. Continue microwaving them in 30-second intervals until they are just a bit runny on top. Then stir with a fork, breaking them apart into large pieces. By the time you "scramble" and stir them, the residual heat should have cooked away the runniness. If they are still undercooked, microwave them on low in 10-second intervals until just done.

Turn the heat under the skillet to low. Stir the eggs into the bacon mixture and season with salt and pepper to taste. Top with the cheese and cover until the cheese melts, 2 to 3 minutes. Transfer to a plate or bowl and serve immediately.

Can be made in 30 minutes or less / No more than 20 minutes hands-on prep time

MAKES 1 SERVING

Each 2-Decadent-Disk serving has: 199 calories, 29 g protein, 10 g carbohydrates, 5 g fat, 2 g saturated fat, 24 mg cholesterol, 2 g fiber, 715 mg sodium

SCRAMBLED EGGS WITH SAUTÉED SHRIMP

2

Years ago, I had brunch at the Bryant Park Grill in New York City. They had the most beautiful and scrumptious dish (I don't remember the exact name, but it was something like Scrambled Eggs with Grilled Jumbo Prawns and Fresh Tomato Slices). They placed a tower of scrambled eggs (or in my case, scrambled egg whites) in the center of the plate. Perfectly grilled jumbo prawns hung from it and fresh tomato slices circled the plate. It was so memorable both because I'd never really realized how much I could enjoy shrimp with eggs and also because it just looked so good. Having thought about how to duplicate it, I created this twist on the flavor combo, and have been in love with it ever since.

Olive oil spray

4 large egg whites

3 ounces medium (31–40 count) raw shrimp, peeled and deveined

$^1/_2$ teaspoon extra virgin olive oil

Salt and pepper

$^3/_4$ teaspoon minced fresh garlic

$^1/_2$ cup fresh pico de gallo or fresh salsa

$1^1/_2$ teaspoons finely chopped fresh cilantro

Lightly mist a medium microwave-safe bowl with spray. Put in the egg whites.

Toss the shrimp with the olive oil and salt and pepper to taste in a small mixing bowl.

Preheat a small nonstick skillet over medium-high heat. Lightly mist the pan with spray. Place the garlic and shrimp in the skillet and cook, stirring frequently, until the shrimp are bright pink and cooked through, 2 to 3 minutes.

Meanwhile, microwave the egg whites on low for 30 seconds. Continue microwaving them in 30-second intervals until they are just a bit runny on top. Then stir with a fork, breaking them apart into large pieces. By the time you "scramble" and stir them, the residual heat should have cooked away the runniness. If they are still undercooked, microwave them on low in 10-second intervals until just done.

Turn the heat under the skillet to low. Gently stir the eggs into the shrimp mixture and stir until well combined. Transfer to a plate or bowl and top with the pico de gallo and cilantro. Season with salt and pepper to taste. Serve immediately.

Can be made in 30 minutes or less / No more than 20 minutes hands-on prep time

MAKES 1 SERVING

2 Each 2-Decadent-Disk serving has: 208 calories, 32 g protein, 10 g carbohydrates, 5 g fat, <1 g saturated fat, 129 mg cholesterol, trace fiber, 408 mg sodium

BACON AND EGG BREAKFAST QUESADILLA

Last year, I was lucky enough to be whisked away to Maui by a guy I was dating. Every morning we'd go to this little café and get the best bacon and egg quesadillas then take them down to the beach. It was pure paradise and inspired this wonderfully decadent dish.

Olive oil spray

4 large egg whites

2 slices center-cut bacon, chopped

2 tablespoons chopped whole green onion

1 (about 8-inch diameter) low-fat, whole-wheat flour tortilla

1 ounce (about $1/2$ cup) finely shredded Cabot's 75% Light Cheddar cheese, or your favorite low-fat Cheddar

1 tablespoon canned chopped mild green chiles, or to taste

Mist a small microwave-safe bowl with spray. Put in the egg whites and set aside.

Place a small nonstick skillet over medium-high heat and put in the bacon. Cook, stirring occasionally, until the bacon is crisp, 5 to 7 minutes. Add the onion and cook until just heated. Remove from the pan and cover to keep warm.

Meanwhile, microwave the egg whites on low for 30 seconds. Continue microwaving them in 30-second intervals until they are just a bit runny on top. Then stir with a fork, breaking them apart into large pieces. By the time you "scramble" and stir them, the residual heat should have cooked away the runniness. If they are still undercooked, microwave them on low in 10-second intervals until just done.

Place a nonstick skillet large enough for the tortilla to lie flat over medium-high heat. Place the tortilla in the pan (no need to add any fat). Sprinkle half of the cheese over half of the tortilla. Then sprinkle the bacon mixture and the chiles over that. Spoon the eggs evenly on top, then sprinkle on the remaining cheese. Fold the bare half over the filled half. Cook for about 2 minutes, until the cheese is beginning to melt and the tortilla is lightly browned in spots. Carefully flip the quesadilla and cook until the cheese is completely melted, another 2 minutes. Serve immediately.

Restaurants typically use very large tortillas for burritos and quesadillas, like the one used in the traditional version of this recipe, which means you eat tons of extra calories and fat. Many store-bought brands are also loaded with fat and are much too big for one person to eat in a sitting.

Can be made in 30 minutes or less / No more than 20 minutes hands-on prep time

MAKES 1 QUESADILLA; 1 SERVING

 Each 3-Decadent-Disk serving (1 quesadilla) has: 298 calories, 30 g protein, 26 g carbohydrates, 9 g fat, 3 g saturated fat, 24 mg cholesterol, 3 g fiber, 829 mg sodium

You save: 433 calories, 31 g fat, 13 g saturated fat, 593 mg sodium

Traditional serving: 731 calories, 30 g protein, 63 g carbohydrates, 40 g fat, 16 g saturated fat, 247 mg cholesterol, 3 g fiber, 1,422 mg sodium

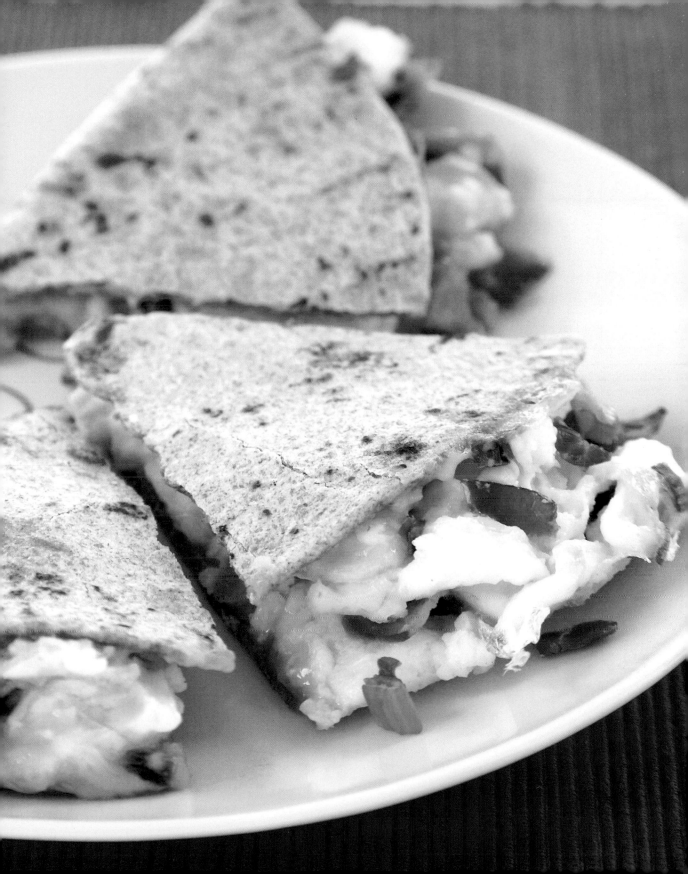

BREAKFAST SAUSAGE LINKS

When I first heard about MySpace (myspace.com), I thought it was for kids and teens. Then when *Fast Food Fix,* my first cookbook, was coming out, my friend Amanda said, "You have to get a MySpace page." Amanda is a voice-over artist and is very tapped in to Hollywood, so I instantly believed her. We put up a page and I started getting all sorts of e-mails and "friend requests" from people who had seen my work. I now love MySpace because so many of my "friends" write and suggest new dishes to create. By far, one of the most requested recipes is breakfast sausage. Obviously everyone loves it. So as a tribute to my MySpace "friends," I created this recipe.

Though I wish I could eliminate even more salt, unfortunately, in this dish, I can't without sacrificing flavor. So don't go crazy eating this every day, especially if your doctor told you to restrict your sodium intake. But it sure will do the trick when the craving for breakfast sausage strikes.

Olive oil spray
$^1/_4$ cup plus 1 tablespoon egg substitute
$^1/_4$ cup plus 1 tablespoon plain dried bread crumbs

$^1/_4$ cup minced sweet onion
1 tablespoon minced fresh garlic
1 teaspoon dried thyme
1 teaspoon black pepper
$^1/_2$ teaspoon dried rosemary
$^1/_2$ teaspoon ground sage
$^1/_2$ teaspoon salt
1 pound extra-lean ground pork

Preheat the oven to 400°F.

Lightly mist a small nonstick baking sheet with spray.

Use a fork to mix the egg substitute, bread crumbs, onion, garlic, thyme, pepper, rosemary, sage, and salt in a medium mixing bowl until well combined. Mix in the pork until well combined. Divide the mixture into 16 equal parts, and then shape each into a 4-inch-long by $^3/_4$-inch-thick link. Place the links side by side, not touching, on the prepared baking sheet. Bake for 5 minutes, then flip and bake for another 3 to 5 minutes, or until no longer pink inside. Serve immediately.

Can be made in 30 minutes or less / No more than 20 minutes hands-on prep time

MAKES 16 LINKS; 8 SERVINGS

Each 1-Decadent-Disk serving (2 links) has: 95 calories, 14 g protein, 4 g carbohydrates, 2 g fat, <1 g saturated fat, 37 mg cholesterol, <1 g fiber, 220 mg sodium

You save (pork sausage): 45 calories, 10 g fat, 4 g saturated fat

You save (turkey sausage): 45 calories, 9 g fat, 3 g saturated fat

Traditional serving (pork sausage): 140 calories, 6 g protein, 1 g carbohydrates, 12 g fat, 4 g saturated fat, 30 mg cholesterol, 0 g fiber, 400 mg sodium

Traditional serving (turkey sausage): 140 calories, 9 g protein, 0 g carbohydrates, 11 g fat, 3 g saturated fat, 45 mg cholesterol, fiber N/A, 360 mg sodium

POTATOES O'BRIEN

❶ ❷

When I was in high school, I had braces (for the second time) and was really fat. I had already missed the junior prom because the only guy I wanted to go with didn't want to go with me. By my senior year, there was one guy who did want to go with me, but he was the only other fat kid in my class. All the kids knew he had asked me, and the teasing began weeks before the big night. Plus I really wasn't interested in him.

So instead, I worked my waitressing job at the Shillington Restaurant. The menu there was very Pennsylvania Dutch. Wednesday nights were smorgasbord nights, my favorite. It was so much easier to wait on a table of buffet eaters than to serve individual entrées. That, and the buffet included the best potatoes O'Brien ever. I looked forward to them every week.

These potatoes are great for dinner, as I was accustomed to eating them back then. But I tend to eat them a lot more as a side with an omelet or scrambled egg whites for breakfast now.

2 small unpeeled baking potatoes (6 ounces each), cut into $^1/_2$-inch cubes
$^3/_4$ cup $^1/_2$-inch onion squares
$^1/_3$ cup drained jarred pimientos
$1^1/_2$ teaspoons extra virgin olive oil
1 teaspoon minced fresh garlic
$^1/_4$ teaspoon paprika
$^1/_8$ teaspoon salt, plus more to taste
Pinch of cayenne
Black pepper

Preheat the oven to 400°F.

Line a medium baking sheet with parchment paper.

Combine the potatoes, onion, pimientos, olive oil, garlic, paprika, $^1/_8$ teaspoon salt, cayenne, and black pepper to taste in a medium glass or plastic mixing bowl. Toss until the potatoes are evenly seasoned, and then transfer the mixture in a single layer to the prepared baking sheet. Bake for 15 minutes, and then flip and bake for another 14 to 18 minutes, until the potatoes are tender when pierced with a knife. Season to taste with additional salt. Serve immediately.

No more than 20 minutes hands-on prep time

MAKES 2 CUPS; 2 SERVINGS OR 4 PORTIONS

❶ Each 1-Decadent-Disk portion ($^1/_2$ cup) has: 101 calories, 2 g protein, 20 g carbohydrates, 2 g fat, trace saturated fat, 0 mg cholesterol, 2 g fiber, 80 mg sodium

❷ Each 2-Decadent-Disk serving (1 cup) has: 201 calories, 5 g protein, 39 g carbohydrates, 4 g fat, <1 g saturated fat, 0 mg cholesterol, 4 g fiber, 160 mg sodium

CHOCOLATE PEANUT BUTTER BREAKFAST "PUDDING"

Okay, okay, so it's not actually pudding. If you want to go get technical on me, it's chocolate peanut butter oatmeal. But imagine my surprise when the combination of these ingredients repeatedly reminded me, and my assistants, of pudding. If you're a big fan of pudding, you're going to love this quick breakfast dish.

A lot of people have trouble having peanut butter in their house. I used to be one of them. If I had a jar in my house, I felt it was practically calling to me when I wasn't even hungry. I've also had a lot of friends who've said it's an addictive food. I still overeat it a tiny bit on occasion, but now that I have such freedom with food, it really isn't a problem. If you can't resist peanut butter, you may want to skip this recipe at first. Then once you're sailing along on *The Most Decadent Diet Ever!* you can definitely reintroduce peanut butter back into your house, and you'll be likely to struggle a lot less with it. If you don't have trouble having it in your house, dig in! You're gonna love this one.

If you prefer natural peanut butter over the reduced-fat version, you can swap that in. Calorie-wise, it's about the same, but you'll be adding a gram of fat and a gram of saturated fat for the 2 teaspoons.

¹/₂ cup old-fashioned rolled oats
1 packet (0.28 g) fat-free, sugar-free hot cocoa mix
2 teaspoons reduced-fat peanut butter
Pinch of salt

Whisk the oats, cocoa mix, peanut butter, salt, and ³/₄ cup water in a medium microwave-safe bowl until well combined. Microwave on high for 2¹/₂ to 3 minutes, or until thickened. Stir and serve immediately.

Can be made in 30 minutes or less / No more than 20 minutes hands-on prep time

MAKES 1 SERVING

Each 3-Decadent-Disk serving has: 305 calories, 12 g protein, 48 g carbohydrates, 7 g fat, 2 g saturated fat, 0 mg cholesterol, 8 g fiber, 349 mg sodium

LEMON-BLUEBERRY OATMEAL

2

We all know that nutritionists, trainers, and often even doctors say that oatmeal is a great breakfast. And we get it. The thing is, if you spend year after year eating the same plain bowl of oatmeal, you're likely to go insane. So I often use the flavors of muffins to inspire new varieties of oatmeal. I've made everything from orange pound cake oatmeal to apple-cinnamon oatmeal, and even a chocolate peanut butter variety (see Chocolate Peanut Butter Breakfast "Pudding," page 46). Now, here's a lemon-blueberry one that is fresh and light in the morning.

Though I have quite the sweet tooth, I've never thought this oatmeal needs much sweetener, so I just added a teaspoon of honey. If you don't agree, feel free to add a packet of artificial sweetener for a no-calorie option. Or add a hint more honey, though that will add 22 calories (0 grams of fat) per teaspoon.

$1/2$ cup old-fashioned rolled oats
$1/2$ teaspoon lemon extract
$1/4$ teaspoon vanilla extract
Pinch of salt
3 tablespoons fresh blueberries or frozen blueberries, defrosted
1 teaspoon honey
1 teaspoon lemon zest
1 packet (0.035 ounce) artificial sweetener, optional

Combine the oats, lemon extract, vanilla, salt, and $3/4$ cup water in a medium microwave-safe bowl. Stir and then microwave on high for $2^1/2$ to 3 minutes, or until thickened. Stir in the blueberries, honey, and lemon zest until well incorporated. Stir in the artificial sweetener, if using. Serve immediately.

Can be made in 30 minutes or less / No more than 20 minutes hands-on prep time

MAKES 1 SERVING

2 Each 2-Decadent-Disk serving has: 206 calories, 7 g protein, 37 g carbohydrates, 3 g fat, trace saturated fat, 0 mg cholesterol, 5 g fiber, 146 mg sodium

BANANA-COCONUT MINI-MUFFINS

I love making mini-muffins because so often I find myself needing just a small treat to satisfy a sweet craving. And because I pride myself on finishing everything I start . . . I joke about that, but I definitely get more pleasure from eating a whole mini-muffin than I do eating half or a third of a standard-sized one.

Same thing with bags of snacks. When I buy cereals or baked chips, I portion them and store them in resealable bags. Then, I put the individual bags back into the bag they came in. By putting the little bags into the bigger bag, I visit the appealing wrapper that, in part, lured me in to begin with. But, even more important, often the bags that chips or cereals come in are designed to keep foods fresh more effectively than resealables. Thus I don't set myself up for potentially stale snacks. When it's time for snacking, I can grab a bag (or sometimes even two) and finish the whole thing(s), just like I can finish these muffins, since they're so small. At only about 50 calories each, one or two of them make the perfect ending to a high-protein, low-fat breakfast. And I can finish every last bite, guilt-free!

Butter-flavored cooking spray
1 cup whole-grain oat flour (see page 17)
$^1/_2$ teaspoon baking soda
$^1/_2$ teaspoon salt
$^1/_4$ teaspoon baking powder

$^1/_2$ cup mashed very ripe banana
$^1/_2$ cup brown sugar (unpacked)
1 large egg white
$^1/_3$ cup fat-free, artificially sweetened vanilla or banana yogurt
$^1/_2$ cup plus 2 tablespoons sweetened flake coconut

Preheat the oven to 350°F.

Mist 18 nonstick mini-muffin cups with spray.

Combine the flour, baking soda, salt, and baking powder in a small bowl. Stir with a fork until combined. Set aside.

Combine the banana, sugar, egg white, and yogurt in a large mixing bowl. Use a sturdy whisk or a spatula to mix until thoroughly blended. Add the flour mixture. Whisk until no flour is visible. Stir in $^1/_2$ cup coconut until evenly distributed in the batter. Then spoon the batter evenly among the prepared muffin cups, filling them three-quarters full. Sprinkle the remaining coconut evenly over the tops.

Bake for 12 to 15 minutes, or until a toothpick inserted in the center comes out dry (a few crumbs are okay).

Cool in the pan on a rack for 10 minutes. Remove the muffins from the pan to the rack and cool completely. Serve warm or at room temperature. Refrigerate any leftovers in an airtight container for up to 3 days.

Can be made in 30 minutes or less / No more than 20 minutes hands-on prep time

MAKES 18 MINI-MUFFINS; 9 SERVINGS

Each 1-Decadent-Disk serving (2 mini-muffins) has: 106 calories, 2 g protein, 20 g carbohydrates, 2 g fat, 1 g saturated fat, trace cholesterol, 2 g fiber, 293 mg sodium

SINLESS YET SINFUL STICKY BUNS

2

Ooey, gooey, and out-of-control drippy! That's what I think of when I think "sticky bun." So how could they be in a diet book? And if they are, how can they be good? Well, rest assured this is a recipe to try. Yes, it takes more time than most others in the book. But even my friends with small children who've never worked with yeast before report having made these over and over. They claim to always be the star of their mommies groups when the other moms learn that these decadent treats are so low in fat and calories. And my friend John, who's quite the bachelor and had never cooked before trying my recipes, had success on the first attempt.

Be careful not to add too much flour to the dough or on your work surface. The dough should stick just a tiny bit so you can roll it out thin. Otherwise, it will bounce back too much. You should, however, definitely flour the rolling pin. You don't want that to stick at all. But please don't let this intimidate you. I promise it really is easy!

1 cup fat-free milk
$^{1}/_{3}$ cup light brown sugar (not packed)
1 tablespoon light butter
$^{1}/_{4}$ cup fat-free, artificially sweetened vanilla yogurt

1 large egg
1 large egg white
1 package ($^{1}/_{4}$ ounce) active dry yeast
$3^{3}/_{4}$ cups plus 4 tablespoons unbleached all-purpose flour, plus more for dusting
$1^{1}/_{2}$ teaspoons ground cinnamon
$^{1}/_{2}$ teaspoon salt
Butter-flavored cooking spray
1 recipe Cinnamon Filling (recipe follows)
1 recipe Sticky Topping (recipe follows)

Combine the milk, brown sugar, and butter in a medium microwave-safe bowl. Microwave on high for about 2 minutes, until the milk is hot (130°F). Whisk in the yogurt and continue whisking until the sugar dissolves (some small lumps of yogurt may be visible). Add the egg and egg white. Whisk to mix well. Add the yeast and whisk in until dissolved.

Combine $3^{3}/_{4}$ cups flour, the cinnamon, and the salt in the bowl of a stand mixer fitted with a dough hook or in a large mixing bowl. Mix with the hook or stir by hand with a wooden spoon. Pour in the milk mixture, and then mix on medium or stir vigorously until well combined. The mixture will be very sticky. One tablespoon at a time, add up to 4 tablespoons of the remaining flour, mixing or stirring to

---

MAKES 20 STICKY BUNS; 20 SERVINGS

2 Each 2-Decadent-Disk serving (1 sticky bun) has: 190 calories, 5 g protein, 37 g carbohydrates, 4 g fat, 2 g saturated fat, 19 mg cholesterol, 1 g fiber, 137 mg sodium
You save: 82 calories, 8 g fat, 2 g saturated fat
Traditional serving: 272 calories, 5 g protein, 38 g carbohydrates, 12 g fat, 4 g saturated fat, 29 mg cholesterol, 1 g fiber, 359 mg sodium

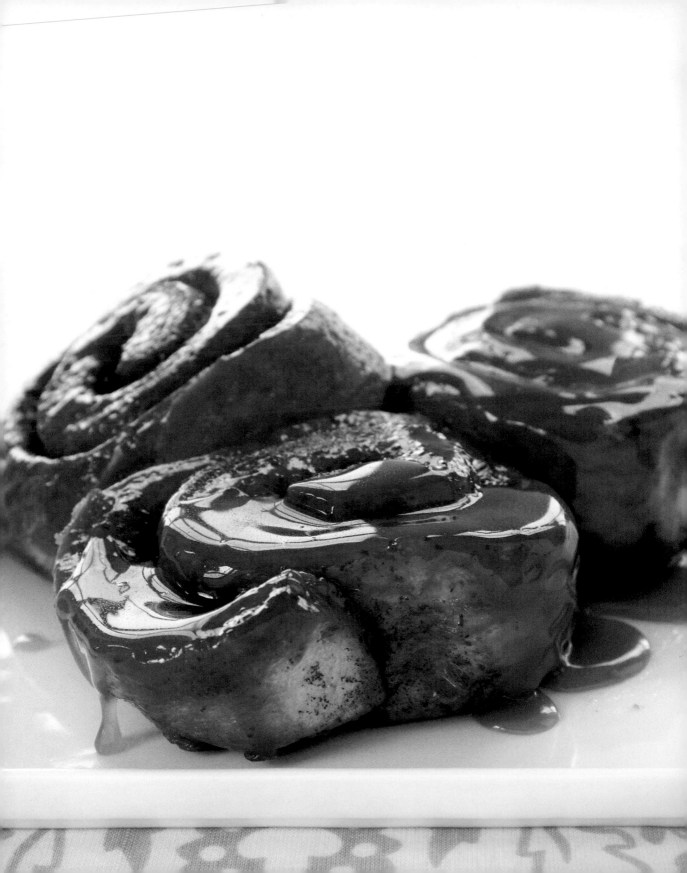

incorporate the flour into the dough until it is just a bit sticky.

Turn the dough onto a floured work surface. Add more flour, no more than 1 tablespoon at a time, if needed, as you knead the dough until it is smooth and elastic, about 5 minutes. The dough should be soft and barely sticky.

Lightly mist a large bowl with spray. Place the dough in the bowl and mist the top of it with spray. Then cover the bowl tightly with plastic wrap. Allow the dough to rise for about 1 hour, or until doubled in size.

Meanwhile, prepare the Cinnamon Filling and the Sticky Topping.

When the dough has doubled, gently punch it down and place it on the lightly floured surface. Knead for 1 minute. Cover with the plastic wrap and allow it to rest for 10 minutes.

Lightly mist a 13 X 9-inch ovenproof glass baking dish with spray. Stir the Sticky Topping just enough to recombine the ingredients, and then pour it into the bottom of the baking dish. Set aside.

Cut the dough in half. Return half of it to the bowl and re-cover it. Use a floured rolling pin (don't reflour the work surface if at all possible) to roll the remaining piece of dough into a 24 X 7-inch rectangle, making sure the ends are as wide and as long as the center. Use a butter knife to spread half of the reserved butter for the Cinnamon Filling evenly over the dough. Sprinkle half of the brown sugar mixture evenly over the top. Starting at one longer side, roll the dough snugly in jelly-roll fashion into a log. Cut the log into 10 equal rounds. Place each round, spiral side up, evenly spaced, in the dish on top of the Sticky Topping. Repeat with the second half of the dough and add the rounds to the dish. Lightly mist a piece of plastic wrap with spray and use it to cover the dish. Refrigerate for 1 hour, or until the sticky buns have risen.

Preheat the oven to 350°F.

Uncover the dish and bake for 21 to 25 minutes, or until just barely golden brown on top and a tiny bit doughy in the very center. Run a butter knife around the sides of the dish to loosen the sticky buns. Turn the hot buns out onto a platter. Cool for about 30 minutes. Brush any of the topping pooling on the platter over the buns, or pull them apart and dip them in it. Serve immediately.

Cinnamon Filling

2 tablespoons light butter
3 tablespoons light brown sugar (packed)
1 1/2 tablespoons ground cinnamon

Place the butter in a small bowl and set it aside to soften. Stir together the brown sugar and cinnamon in a second small bowl.

Sticky Topping

1/4 cup light brown sugar (packed)
1/2 cup light butter, room temperature
3 tablespoons honey
1/3 cup dark corn syrup

Use an electric mixer fitted with beaters to beat the brown sugar, butter, honey, and corn syrup in a medium mixing bowl until well combined.

BANANA COLADA SMOOTHIE

🟊1🟊 🟊2🟊

I'm a big fan of the piña colada, as is my mother. I started ordering virgins when I was a little kid, following my mother's example. Little did I know in my youth that they are full of heavy cream and other potentially hip-expanding ingredients. This is one of my adult tributes to them. It's a great breakfast treat or a refreshing afternoon snack.

1 cup frozen pineapple chunks or tidbits
$^1/_2$ small ripe banana
$^1/_4$ cup light coconut milk
$^1/_4$ cup fat-free milk
$^1/_4$ cup fat-free, artificially sweetened vanilla
    yogurt

Place all of the ingredients in the jar of a blender with ice-crushing ability. Make sure the lid is on tight. Use the "purée" or "ice crush" setting to blend the ingredients until they are relatively smooth. Then blend on the "liquefy" or "high speed" setting for a few seconds, until completely smooth. Transfer to a glass and serve immediately.

Can be made in 30 minutes or less / No more than 20 minutes hands-on prep time

MAKES 14 OUNCES; 1 SERVING OR 2 PORTIONS

🟊1🟊 Each 1-Decadent-Disk portion (about 7 ounces) has: 104 calories, 3 g protein, 21 g carbohydrates, 2 g fat, 2 g saturated fat, 1 mg cholesterol, 2 g fiber, 35 mg sodium

🟊2🟊 Each 2-Decadent-Disk serving (about 14 ounces) has: 209 calories, 5 g protein, 41 g carbohydrates, 4 g fat, 3 g saturated fat, 3 mg cholesterol, 3 g fiber, 71 mg sodium

CINNAMON APPLE YOGURT PARFAIT

2

It's always hard to get your "five-a-day," isn't it? We want to go for the cookie or the brownie, and I'm all for that, but not instead of the good-for-you (or me!) stuff. One of the ways I really enjoy fruit is to dip it in fat-free vanilla yogurt spiked with a bit of cinnamon. Here's a fun enhancement of that concept that can be made really festive if served in a wineglass or other fancy glass.

I created this recipe using artificially sweetened yogurt because the client I originally made it for cares more about food being as low in calories as possible than she does about it being all-natural. If you don't want to eat the artificially sweetened varieties, you can substitute one sweetened with sugar or honey, but those will add 70 to 80 calories and 2 grams of fat to this parfait.

²/₃ cup fat-free, artificially sweetened vanilla yogurt
¹/₄ to ¹/₂ teaspoon ground cinnamon
¹/₃ cup bite-sized apple pieces
4 tablespoons low-fat granola without raisins, divided

Mix the yogurt and cinnamon in a small bowl until well combined. Spoon half of the yogurt mixture into a wineglass. Sprinkle half of the apple pieces evenly over the top of the yogurt mixture, followed by 2 tablespoons granola. Repeat with the remaining ingredients. Serve immediately.

Can be made in 30 minutes or less / No more than 20 minutes hands-on prep time

MAKES 1 PARFAIT; 1 SERVING

2 Each 2-Decadent-Disk serving (1 parfait) has: 208 calories, 7 g protein, 42 g carbohydrates, 1 g fat, trace saturated fat, 3 mg cholesterol, 3 g fiber, 155 mg sodium

WHAT IF THE SAYING WENT "A burger a day keeps the doctor away"? Pretty cool, huh? Well, I'm going to argue that burgers, a few sandwiches, and some wraps very well could. I'm not suggesting you grab your keys and head for the local burger joint or sandwich shop. And I'm not about to serve up recipe after recipe of veggie burgers to prove my point. I'm suggesting that my style of cooking lends itself to indulging in our favorites without paying a price.

Here's a chapter full of moderate-sized, decadent burgers, sandwiches, and wraps to start you on your quest to enjoying "real food" the way you love it, in a healthier way. If you couple these sandwiches with some slightly less decadent, yet still delicious ones from time to time (filled with lean meats and veggies stacked on whole-grain breads), your doctor is definitely likely to wonder what your secret is.

I sort of think of burgers, sandwiches, and wraps as "rescue me" foods. They're so easy to throw together (yes, a few of the ultra-decadent ones featured here are a bit more time consuming, but you can tweak them slightly to put them together in minutes). They rescued me from spending too much money on lunch when I was working in an office. They rescue me when I just don't feel like cooking and I need a hearty meal. And they rescue me when I want a lazy meal for entertaining. Who doesn't love a burger buffet? If you ask me, burgers just may be the perfect food.

3 Blue Cheese Mushroom Burger

3 BBQ Bacon Cheeseburger

3 Present-Day Patty Melt

2 Chunky-No-More Chili Dog

2 Bacon Cheese Dog

3 Greek Isle Pocket

3 Sexier Sausage and Pepper Sub

1 **2** **4** Health Club Sandwich

3 Turkey Sandwich with Cranberry Aioli

3 Muscles Meatloaf Sandwich

3 Roasted Pork Sandwich

3 Crispy Bacon Chicken Breast Sandwich

3 Warm Brie Chicken Breast Sandwich

3 Hotter Turkey Sandwich

4 Curry Chicken Wrap

3 Open-Face Ham and Cheese

3 Gourmet Roast Beef Pocket

3 Open-Ended Buffalo Chicken Wrap

3 Renovated Reuben Wrap

BLUE CHEESE MUSHROOM BURGER

③

I always say that the sign of a good burger is whether you need a napkin to eat it. People often comment (before sampling my burgers, of course) that the leanest cuts of beef are dry. Not true. If you cook and season this burger properly (whatever you do, make sure your pan is nice and hot before you put the burger in it) and you don't smash it with a spatula, you're guaranteed a juicy, drippy burger.

One of the reasons I love blue cheese so much is that it packs such strong flavor—you only ever need a little bit. Now that I've found a reduced-fat variety, I'm even happier. I buy Treasure Cave brand. One ounce has 81 calories and 5 grams of fat. If you have trouble finding it and want to substitute $^3/_4$ ounce of the full-fat variety, that will add 20 calories and 3 grams of fat to this dish.

$3^1/_2$ ounces 96% lean ground beef
$^3/_4$ ounce (about 3 tablespoons) crumbled reduced-fat blue cheese
Salt and pepper
Garlic powder
Olive oil spray
$^1/_2$ cup sliced button mushrooms
1 whole-wheat or whole-grain hamburger bun

Divide the beef in half and shape each into a ball, packing each tightly. On a sheet of wax paper, press each ball into a 4-inch-diameter patty. Sprinkle the cheese evenly over the center of one patty, leaving the outer $^1/_2$ inch uncovered. Place the second patty on top of the first and seal the edges well. Sprinkle both sides of the stuffed patty lightly with salt, pepper, and garlic powder to taste.

Lightly mist a medium nonstick skillet with spray and place it over medium-high heat. Put in the mushrooms and cook, stirring occasionally, until tender and lightly browned on the outsides, 3 to 5 minutes. Season with salt, pepper, and garlic powder to taste. Transfer the mushrooms to a small covered bowl to keep them warm.

Return the skillet to the heat. When it is hot, place the patty on one side of the pan, and then place the bun halves, insides facedown, next to the patty. Cook the patty for 1 to 2 minutes per side for medium-rare, or until the desired doneness is reached. Cook the bun halves until just toasted, 1 to 2 minutes.

Place the bun bottom on a serving plate. Add the patty to the toasted bun bottom. Mound the mushrooms on top. Place the bun top atop the sandwich. Serve immediately.

Can be made in 30 minutes or less / No more than 20 minutes hands-on prep time

MAKES 1 BURGER; 1 SERVING

③ Each 3-Decadent-Disk serving (1 burger) has: 299 calories, 29 g protein, 24 g carbohydrates, 10 g fat, 4 g saturated fat, 64 mg cholesterol, 4 g fiber, 553 mg sodium

You save: 49 calories, 11 g fat, 4 g saturated fat

Traditional serving: 348 calories, 27 g protein, 20 g carbohydrates, 21 g fat, 8 g saturated fat, 81 mg cholesterol, 2 g fiber, 765 mg sodium

BBQ Bacon Cheeseburger with Italian Seasoned Fries (page 166)

BBQ BACON CHEESEBURGER

3

The barbecue bacon cheeseburger is usually a guilty pleasure. Here, I've combined these favorite flavors in a reasonable-sized burger that's even more scrumptious because the ingredients are fresh and guilt free. Please, though, don't cheat when buying the beef. Some people think that buying 93% lean ground beef isn't that much different from the 96% lean, but it is. Four ounces of the 96% lean has about 150 calories and 4^1/$_2$ grams of fat. Four ounces of the 93% lean has 170 calories and 8 grams of fat. Yes, the 96% lean is more expensive, but you're worth it (plus, in the long term, you'll be saving money on doctor bills)!

4 ounces 96% lean ground beef
Pinch of salt
1^1/$_2$ slices center-cut bacon
1 reduced-calorie hamburger bun
^{1}/$_2$ ounce light Swiss cheese slivers
1 to 2 tablespoons red onion slivers
2 teaspoons barbecue sauce

Pack the beef tightly together with your hands, and then shape it into a 4-inch-diameter patty on a sheet of wax paper. Sprinkle lightly with salt on both sides, and then place in the freezer for 5 minutes (to help the patty keep its shape).

Preheat a grill to high.

Cut the whole bacon strip in half crosswise. Lay the 3 half strips side by side in a small nonstick skillet over medium heat. Cook, flipping them every couple of minutes, until crispy and well done, 6 to 8 minutes. Transfer the bacon to a paper towel–lined plate to drain.

Meanwhile, remove the patty from the freezer and place it on the grill. Cook for 1 to 2 minutes per side for medium rare, or until the desired doneness is reached. Toast the bun halves on an upper grill rack for 30 seconds to 1 minute, watching them carefully. Place the cheese on top of the burger for the last few seconds of cooking so it just begins to melt.

Add the patty to the toasted bun bottom. Lay the bacon strips side by side over the top. Place the onion over that. Spread the barbecue sauce evenly over the inside of the top half of the bun. Place the bun top atop the sandwich. Serve immediately.

Can be made in 30 minutes or less / No more than 20 minutes hands-on prep time

MAKES 1 BURGER; 1 SERVING

3 Each 3-Decadent-Disk serving (1 burger) has: 304 calories, 33 g protein, 23 g carbohydrates, 10 g fat, 4 g saturated fat, 75 mg cholesterol, 3 g fiber, 752 mg sodium

You save: 180 calories, 22 g fat, 8 g saturated fat

Traditional serving: 484 calories, 29 g protein, 19 g carbohydrates, 32 g fat, 12 g saturated fat, 99 mg cholesterol, 1 g fiber, 712 mg sodium

PRESENT-DAY PATTY MELT

3

No matter where you order them, patty melts can never be the leanest item on the menu. After all, patty melts are beef with two kinds of cheese and they're one of the few sandwiches that require at least a little bit of fat on the outside of the bread. This modified version, however, is sure to curb the craving when it hits. And the good news is that it won't set you back the way the restaurant versions will.

3 ounces 96% lean ground beef

2 pinches of garlic powder

Salt and pepper

2 teaspoons light butter, divided

2 slices light multigrain or seven-grain bread

Olive oil spray

$^1/_4$ cup onion slivers

$^1/_2$ ounce light Swiss cheese slivers

$^1/_2$ ounce (about $^1/_4$ cup) Cabot's 75% Light Cheddar cheese slivers, or your favorite low-fat Cheddar

1 tablespoon ketchup, optional

Place a sheet of wax paper on a flat work surface. Press the beef into a ball, packing it tightly. Then transfer it to the wax paper and press it out so that it is about $^1/_2$ inch longer and wider than the bread slices (it will be very thin). Season the top of the patty with a pinch of garlic powder and salt and pepper to taste, and then place it in the freezer for 5 minutes (to help it keep its shape).

Spread 1 teaspoon butter over one side of each slice of bread.

Place a medium nonstick skillet over medium heat. Mist it with spray and put in the onions. Cook until tender but not browned, 5 to 7 minutes. Transfer to a plate and cover to keep them warm. Turn the heat to medium-high. When the skillet is hot, transfer the patty into the skillet. Season the second side with the remaining garlic powder and salt and pepper to taste. Cook for 1 to 2 minutes per side, or until the desired doneness is reached.

Add the patty to the plate with the onions and cover.

Turn the heat to medium. Place one slice of bread, buttered side down, in the skillet. Top it evenly with the Swiss cheese. Place the second slice, buttered side down, next to the first. Add the Cheddar slivers evenly over that. Top the Cheddar with the patty, followed by the onion. Add ketchup, if desired. When the Swiss cheese is almost melted and the bread is golden brown, place the slice with the Swiss cheese on top of the sandwich. Press down with a spatula. Serve immediately.

Can be made in 30 minutes or less / No more than 20 minutes hands-on prep time

MAKES 1 SANDWICH; 1 SERVING

3 Each 3-Decadent-Disk serving (1 sandwich) has: 309 calories, 30 g protein, 23 g carbohydrates, 11 g fat, 5 g saturated fat, 65 mg cholesterol, 2 g fiber, 474 mg sodium

You save: 145 calories, 23 g fat, 14 g saturated fat

Traditional serving: 454 calories, 20 g protein, 19 g carbohydrates, 34 g fat, 19 g saturated fat, 104 mg cholesterol, 2 g fiber, 501 mg sodium

CHUNKY-NO-MORE CHILI DOG

2

Have you ever tried a fat-free hot dog? I know, they don't sound like they would be great, but some brands really are, especially when you add things like bacon and cheese (see the Bacon Cheese Dog, page 60) and chili. You can even make excellent pigs-in-a-blanket with them using low-fat biscuit dough. I serve those to my friends all the time, and as long as I cover them completely in the dough (completely enclosing them ensures that the dogs stay juicy), no one ever knows the difference. This chili dog is another example of how great a low-fat, low-calorie meal (or even snack) can be. With only 203 calories, this has about the same number of calories as a small protein bar, and you can bet it's a whole lot more filling. Granted, these dogs are a little high in sodium, so you don't want to eat them too often, but with 5 grams of fiber, they sure are a worthy craving-buster.

One 97% fat-free or fat-free beef or turkey hot dog
3 tablespoons Chipotle Chili without the blue cheese (page 129), reheated if necessary
1 whole-grain hot dog bun

Half-fill a small nonstick saucepan with water. Place the pan over high heat and bring the water to a boil. Add the hot dog and cook, uncovered, until heated through and plumped slightly, about 3 minutes.

Meanwhile, place a small nonstick skillet over medium heat. Open the bun and place it, inside facedown, in the skillet and cook until the inside is lightly toasted, 3 to 5 minutes. Transfer the bun to a plate.

Place the cooked hot dog in the bun. Top the dog evenly with the chili. Serve immediately.

Can be made in 30 minutes or less / No more than 20 minutes hands-on prep time

MAKES 1 CHILI DOG; 1 SERVING

2 Each 2-Decadent-Disk serving (1 chili dog) has: 203 calories, 15 g protein, 30 g carbohydrates, 4 g fat, 1 g saturated fat, 22 mg cholesterol, 5 g fiber, 715 mg sodium

You save: 87 calories, 9 g fat, 3 g saturated fat

Traditional serving: 290 calories, 11 g protein, 31 g carbohydrates, 13 g fat, 4 g saturated fat, 30 mg cholesterol, 1 g fiber, 1,000 mg sodium

BACON CHEESE DOG

2

When I was a kid, I learned to make the full-fat variety of these dogs, and boy were they tasty. Amazingly, so is this low-fat version. But what is more amazing is that the whole thing is a mere 203 calories! This is, of course, another dish where I just could not remove as much sodium as I'd like (how can you remove sodium from a hot dog or strip of bacon?), so don't overindulge. However, here's more proof that you can eat almost anything you love, even when living a healthy lifestyle.

One 97% fat-free or fat-free beef or turkey hot dog

$^1/_3$ ounce (about 3 tablespoons) shredded Cabot's 75% Light Cheddar cheese, or your favorite low-fat Cheddar

1 slice center-cut bacon

1 whole-wheat or whole-grain hot dog bun

Preheat the oven to 450°F.

Place a metal baking rack on top of a baking sheet of approximately the same size.

Cut a slit down the length of the hot dog, cutting about two-thirds of the way into the dog. Fill the slit with the cheese, and then wrap the bacon on a diagonal around the dog, covering as much surface area as possible. Secure the ends with toothpicks to keep the bacon and cheese in place. Place the dog on the baking rack with the cheese facing up and bake for 13 to 15 minutes, or until the bacon is starting to crisp and the cheese is melted.

During the last few minutes of cooking the dog, toast the bun, if desired, in the oven by placing it, inside facedown, on the baking rack for 2 to 3 minutes, until toasted. Transfer the bun to a plate. Place the dog in the bun and serve immediately.

Can be made in 30 minutes or less / No more than 20 minutes hands-on prep time

MAKES 1 CHEESE DOG; 1 SERVING

2 Each 2-Decadent-Disk serving (1 cheese dog) has: 203 calories, 15 g protein, 25 g carbohydrates, 6 g fat, 3 g saturated fat, 25 mg cholesterol, 3 g fiber, 797 mg sodium

You save: 238 calories, 25 g fat, 10 g saturated fat

Traditional serving: 441 calories, 15 g protein, 25 g carbohydrates, 31 g fat, 13 g saturated fat, 61 mg cholesterol, <1 g fiber, 1,075 mg sodium

GREEK ISLE POCKET

3

Mediterranean Layer Dip is one of my all-time favorite appetizers to serve at parties. For years there was rarely any left over, so I started making more and more because I loved having it the next day as a spread or in a sandwich. Here's a super-easy treat for any leftovers you might have.

You can use grilled chicken purchased at the grocery store to make this dish even simpler; just be mindful of the sodium. Some brands tend to be laden with salt.

1 (about 6½-inch diameter) whole-wheat pita circle
¼ cup plus 2 tablespoons Mediterranean Layer Dip (page 197)
4 ounces sliced Basic Grilled Chicken (recipe follows) or other extra-lean grilled chicken breast

Place the pita on a cutting board. Cut off a third of it and reserve for another use, such as for dipping with Bacon Horseradish Dip (page 205) or Mediterranean Layer Dip. Open the pita just enough to spread the dip evenly inside. Add the chicken slices. Serve immediately or wrap in plastic and refrigerate for up to 4 hours.

BASIC GRILLED CHICKEN

1 pound boneless, skinless chicken breast, visible fat removed
1 teaspoon extra virgin olive oil
Salt and pepper

Preheat a grill to high.

Rub the chicken breast with olive oil and season both sides with salt and pepper to taste. Transfer to the grill and cook for 3 to 5 minutes per side, or until no longer pink inside.

Makes 4 chicken breasts; 4 servings
Each serving has: 135 calories, 26 g protein, 0 g carbohydrates, 3 g fat, 1 g saturated fat, 66 mg cholesterol, 0 g fiber, 74 mg sodium

---

MAKES 1 POCKET; 1 SERVING

3 Each 3-Decadent-Disk serving (1 pita pocket) has: 296 calories, 34 g protein, 24 g carbohydrates, 8 g fat, 2 g saturated fat, 69 mg cholesterol, 4 g fiber, 546 mg sodium

SEXIER SAUSAGE AND PEPPER SUB

3

The classic "hoagie shop" sausage and pepper sub is one of the sandwiches I most miss from my Pennsylvania childhood. When I make this sandwich, I always use a 6-inch piece of whole-grain French baguette. I could use a sub roll, but they're so wide, the piece would be too short. Instead, I cut a 6-inch piece of baguette, then weigh it. If it's 2 ounces, I keep it as is. If not, I pull out enough of the inside, being careful not to tear the outside, so that it weighs only 2 ounces. The finished sandwich looks bigger and I get a great protein-to-carb ratio.

Olive oil spray

$1/2$ recipe Sweet and Slim Italian Sausage, unshaped and uncooked (page 130)

One 6-ounce piece (about 18 inches) of a multigrain or whole-wheat French baguette

$1^1/3$ cups onion strips (roughly 3 inches long, $1/4$ inch thick)

$1/2$ cup green bell pepper strips (roughly 3 inches long, $1/4$ inch thick; see page 20)

Salt and pepper

Crushed red pepper flakes

2 teaspoons sliced, pickled hot chiles, or more to taste, optional

Preheat the oven to 400°F.

Mist a small nonstick baking sheet with spray.

Shape the Sweet and Slim Italian Sausage mixture into 3 links that are each $6^1/2$ inches long. Place the links side by side, not touching, on the prepared baking sheet. Bake for 10 to 13 minutes, or until no longer pink inside.

Cut the baguette into 3 equal pieces, each about 6 inches long. Then cut them lengthwise just enough so they will open. Wrap them in a sheet of aluminum foil large enough to cover them completely. Heat in the oven for 8 to 10 minutes, until warm inside and the outsides just begin to crisp slightly.

Place a medium nonstick skillet over medium-high heat. When the skillet is hot, mist it with spray, and then put in the onion and bell pepper. Cook, stirring occasionally until lightly browned, for about 3 minutes, and then turn the heat to medium and cook until completely tender, 3 to 5 minutes. Season with salt, pepper, and red pepper flakes to taste.

Weigh the baguettes, if possible. If they weigh more than 2 ounces each, carefully pull enough dough from the centers, without tearing the outsides, so that they weigh 2 ounces. Place each baguette on a plate. Add 1 sausage link to each, and then top each with a third of the onion mixture and a third of the chiles. Serve immediately.

Can be made in 30 minutes or less

MAKES 3 SANDWICHES; 3 SERVINGS

3 Each 3-Decadent-Disk serving (1 sandwich) has: 306 calories, 24 g protein, 40 g carbohydrates, 5 g fat, <1 g saturated fat, 49 mg cholesterol, 4 g fiber, 626 mg sodium

You save: 309 calories, 21 g fat, 11 g saturated fat

Traditional serving: 615 calories, 29 g protein, 82 g carbohydrates, 26 g fat, 11 g saturated fat, 41 mg cholesterol, 6 g fiber, 1,890 mg sodium

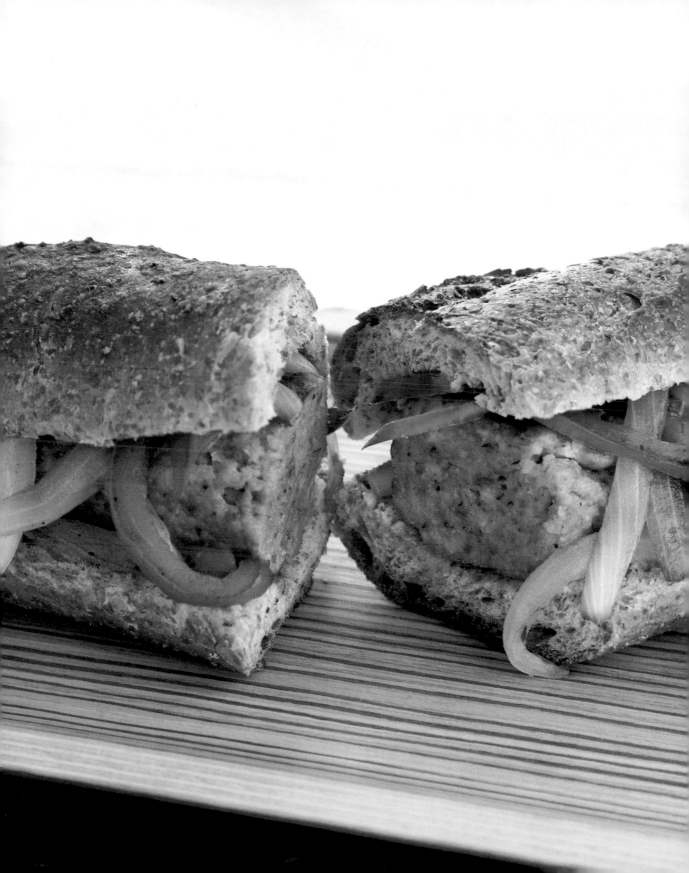

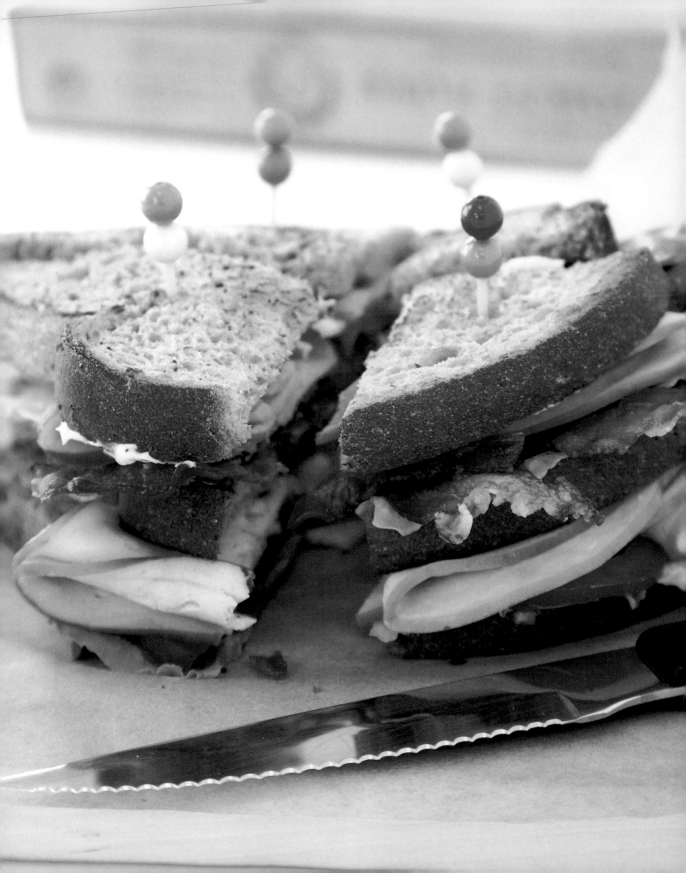

HEALTH CLUB SANDWICH

1 2 4

Any time I see a club sandwich, I think of my mother. When I was a kid, my mom always ordered them, while I ordered chicken parmesan sandwiches wherever we were. At the time, I never got the appeal of a club—why would one eat turkey, when you could be eating something fried and dripping with cheese? Now I love them. Back then, I found it fascinating that my mother could eat just one or two quarters as her entire meal. These days, I often eat just two quarters, but I always eat them with a small salad or follow them with a piece of fruit or some On-the-Terrace Fruit Salad (page 222).

2 slices center-cut bacon, cut in half
3 slices light wheat bread
1 tablespoon light mayonnaise
1 romaine lettuce leaf
4 slices Roma tomato
Salt and pepper
5 ounces thinly sliced extra-lean roasted turkey or
    extra-lean shaved deli turkey

Place a small nonstick skillet over medium-high heat. Add the bacon and cook until crisp, about 5 minutes. Transfer the bacon to a paper towel–lined plate to drain. Just before the bacon is cooked, toast the bread slices until lightly toasted on both sides. Then place them side by side on a clean work surface. Spread 1/2 teaspoons mayonnaise on the first and third slices of bread. Place the lettuce and then the tomato on the first slice. Season with salt and pepper to taste. Top evenly with half of the turkey. Top that with the bare slice of bread. Add the remaining turkey, followed by the bacon. Place the remaining slice of bread atop the sandwich. Secure the sandwich layers together by piercing them through the top bread slice with 4 decorative toothpicks placed in a diamond pattern so they go all of the way through the sandwich. Use a serrated knife to cut the sandwich diagonally into 4 triangles (a toothpick should be securing each quarter). Serve immediately.

The *Most Decadent Diet Ever!* version of this sandwich has lots of protein for a more satisfying and healthier meal than the traditional club, which provides tons of fat and very little protein.

Can be made in 30 minutes or less / No more than 20 minutes hands-on prep time

MAKES 1 SANDWICH; 1 SERVING OR 2 OR 4 PORTIONS

1 Each 1-Decadent-Disk portion (1/4 sandwich) has: 98 calories, 11 g protein, 8 g carbohydrates, 3 g fat, <1 g saturated fat, 18 mg cholesterol, 3 g fiber, 273 mg sodium

2 Each 2-Decadent-Disk portion (1/2 sandwich) has: 196 calories, 22 g protein, 16 g carbohydrates, 6 g fat, 1 g saturated fat, 36 mg cholesterol, 6 g fiber, 547 mg sodium

4 Each 4-Decadent-Disk serving (1 sandwich) has: 393 calories, 45 g protein, 33 g carbohydrates, 11 g fat, 3 g saturated fat, 73 mg cholesterol, 12 g fiber, 1,093 mg sodium

You save: 157 calories, 21 g fat, 2 g saturated fat

Traditional serving: 550 calories, 24 g protein, 39 g carbohydrates, 32 g fat, 5 g saturated fat, 55 mg cholesterol, 3 g fiber, 1,600 mg sodium

TURKEY SANDWICH WITH CRANBERRY AIOLI

My cousin Cathie called me recently and told me that her new favorite sandwich to take to work for lunch was turkey with lettuce, cranberry sauce, and mayonnaise. She thought I should consider putting it in my book. Though I get great suggestions from my friends and fans, in this case, I beat her to the punch. I often make this sandwich the day after Thanksgiving or any other day of the year with leftovers from Sage Butter Roasted Turkey (page 148), and it is heaven. Or if I don't have any turkey leftovers on hand, I'll just grab some turkey at the deli counter at my local grocery store. Be careful if you do that, though, because many brands can be insanely high in sodium.

You'll notice throughout the book that there are times when I use light mayonnaise and others when I use low-fat. It's not a mistake. I stock both in my refrigerator. Low-fat mayonnaise has about 25 calories and 2 grams of fat per tablespoon, while the light one has 45 calories and 5 grams of fat per tablespoon. The light one tastes closer to traditional mayonnaise, so when I'm really using it to flavor something like this sandwich, which contains mild flavors, I use light. If I'm using stronger flavors, as in the Curry Chicken Wrap (page 73), I use the low-fat. In those, it's needed only for texture.

1 tablespoon cranberry sauce
$1^1/_2$ teaspoons light mayonnaise
$^1/_4$ teaspoon dried rosemary, or more to taste
2 slices whole-grain bread
$3^3/_4$ ounces extra-lean shaved turkey (low-sodium preferred)
1 leaf red or green leaf lettuce

Whisk the cranberry sauce, mayonnaise, and rosemary in a small bowl, until smooth and well combined.

Place one slice of bread on a plate. Pile the turkey evenly on top of it. Add the lettuce. Spread the cranberry mixture evenly over the second slice of bread, and then flip the slice atop the sandwich. Serve immediately, or wrap tightly in plastic wrap and refrigerate until ready to serve.

Although I did not find direct comparatives for this recipe, I came across a few recipes for basic turkey sandwiches with as much as 38 grams of fat per serving and 1,900 mg sodium!

Can be made in 30 minutes or less / No more than 20 minutes hands-on prep time

MAKES 1 SANDWICH; 1 SERVING

Each 3-Decadent-Disk serving (1 sandwich) has: 304 calories, 31 g protein, 32 mg carbohydrates, 6 g fat, <1 g saturated fat, 44 mg cholesterol, 4 g fiber, 589 mg sodium

MUSCLES MEATLOAF SANDWICH

3

My friend Nick is a huge fan of meatloaf. When I was working on developing various meatloaves last year, he had me take field trips of sorts to some of his favorite meatloaf stops around Los Angeles. I was fascinated by all the different varieties and astounded by how much fat and how many calories most have. After I ran through all of my trials, Nick stopped by for the leftovers. Apparently, he loves meatloaf sandwiches, too. This was his favorite.

2 slices whole-grain bread
1¹/₂ slices (³/₄ serving) Mini-Meatloaves (page 128)
¹/₂ leaf green leaf lettuce
2 teaspoons to 1 tablespoon lower-sodium ketchup

Place one slice of bread on a plate. Top it evenly with the meatloaf slices, followed by the lettuce. Spread the ketchup on the remaining slice of bread and flip it atop the sandwich. Serve immediately, or wrap in plastic wrap and refrigerate for up to 6 hours.

Can be made in 30 minutes or less / No more than 20 minutes hands-on prep time

MAKES 1 SANDWICH; 1 SERVING

3 Each 3-Decadent-Disk serving (1 sandwich) has: 298 calories, 25 g protein, 38 g carbohydrates, 6 g fat, 2 g saturated fat, 45 mg cholesterol, 5 g fiber, 537 mg sodium

You save: 117 calories, 11 g fat, 4 g saturated fat

Traditional serving: 415 calories, 28 g protein, 37 g carbohydrates, 17 g fat, 6 g saturated fat, 79 mg cholesterol, fiber N/A, 526 mg sodium

ROASTED PORK SANDWICH

3

I had an ex-boyfriend who never let me watch healthy cooking shows at night. He said that watching me was like watching a guy watch a football game. I would get so into the shows and often was so disappointed. One night, I was watching an episode of a show where the host made pulled "pork" out of turkey legs (there was no pork in the dish at all!). I got pretty animated; "Are you kidding me?!" I yelled at the TV. I knew that the leanest cut of pork has $3^1/2$ grams of fat for a 4-ounce serving, and a 4-ounce serving of turkey leg meat has 5 grams of fat. But the last straw was when, on another episode, he made a Philly cheesesteak open-face and out of turkey legs! Using methods like substituting turkey for pork, which is so different in flavor, texture, and so on, is exactly how the media create the impression that healthy food doesn't taste great. So here's a pork sandwich with—you guessed it—real pork. I bet you won't be disappointed, especially since it's way leaner.

2 slices whole-grain bread

$3^3/4$ ounces Honey-Glazed Spiced Pork Tenderloin (page 126), or other extra-lean roasted pork, sliced very thin

$^1/4$ cup Colorful Coleslaw (page 189) or other low-fat coleslaw

Place one slice of bread on a plate. Mound the pork evenly over it. Spoon the coleslaw evenly over the pork and place the second slice of bread atop the sandwich. Cut in half and serve immediately, or wrap in plastic wrap and refrigerate for up to 8 hours.

MAKES 1 SANDWICH; 1 SERVING

3 Each 3-Decadent-Disk serving (1 sandwich) has: 305 calories, 27 g protein, 33 g carbohydrates, 8 g fat, 2 g saturated fat, 65 mg cholesterol, 5 g fiber, 587 mg sodium

CRISPY BACON CHICKEN BREAST SANDWICH

Part of what I love about a chicken breast sandwich is its versatility. You can grill chicken breasts and then add all sorts of toppings to make new meals every day. I love simply throwing a bit of lettuce, tomato, onion, and barbecue sauce on them or adding some sautéed onions and mushrooms, or even a bit of low-fat marinara sauce and some low-fat mozzarella to create a chicken parmesan sandwich.

But here is a classic combo of bacon and Swiss that we Americans tend to love. Feel free to stick to this version or to come up with your own favorite ingredient combos. The base of just the chicken breast and the whole-grain hamburger bun has 210 calories and 3 grams of fat.

One 3-ounce boneless, skinless chicken breast, visible fat removed
Olive oil spray
Salt and pepper
1^1/$_2$ slices center-cut bacon
^{1}/$_2$ ounce light Swiss cheese shavings
1 whole-grain hamburger bun
1 leaf green-leaf lettuce
Two ^{1}/$_4$-inch tomato slices
1 teaspoon light mayonnaise

Preheat a grill to high.

Place the chicken breast between two sheets of plastic wrap or wax paper on a flat work surface. Use the flat side of a meat mallet to pound it to an even thickness, about ^{1}/$_2$ inch. Lightly mist with spray, and then sprinkle with salt and pepper to taste.

Cut the whole bacon strip in half crosswise. Lay the 3 half strips side by side in a small nonstick skillet over medium-high heat. Cook for 2 to 4 minutes per side, until crispy. Transfer the bacon to a paper towel-lined plate to drain.

Meanwhile, place the chicken on the grill. Turn the heat to medium, if possible, and cook for 3 to 5 minutes per side, until no longer pink inside. During the last minute, add the cheese to the chicken and place the bun, insides facedown, on a top grill rack to toast, if desired.

Place the bun bottom, inside faceup, on a plate. Add the chicken breast and then the bacon strips, side by side, the lettuce, and the tomato slices. Spread the mayonnaise evenly over the inside of the bun top and place it on top of the sandwich. Serve immediately.

The "fast-food" version of this sandwich uses a huge bun that adds tons of calories and carbs with few nutrients.

Can be made in 30 minutes or less / No more than 20 minutes hands-on prep time

MAKES 1 SANDWICH; 1 SERVING

Each 3-Decadent-Disk serving (1 sandwich) has: 304 calories, 32 g protein, 22 g carbohydrates, 10 g fat, 3 g saturated fat, 66 mg cholesterol, 2 g fiber, 550 mg sodium

You save: 246 calories, 15 g fat, 4 g saturated fat

Traditional serving: 550 calories, 40 g protein, 43 g carbohydrates, 25 g fat, 7 g saturated fat, 95 mg cholesterol, fiber N/A, 1,410 mg sodium

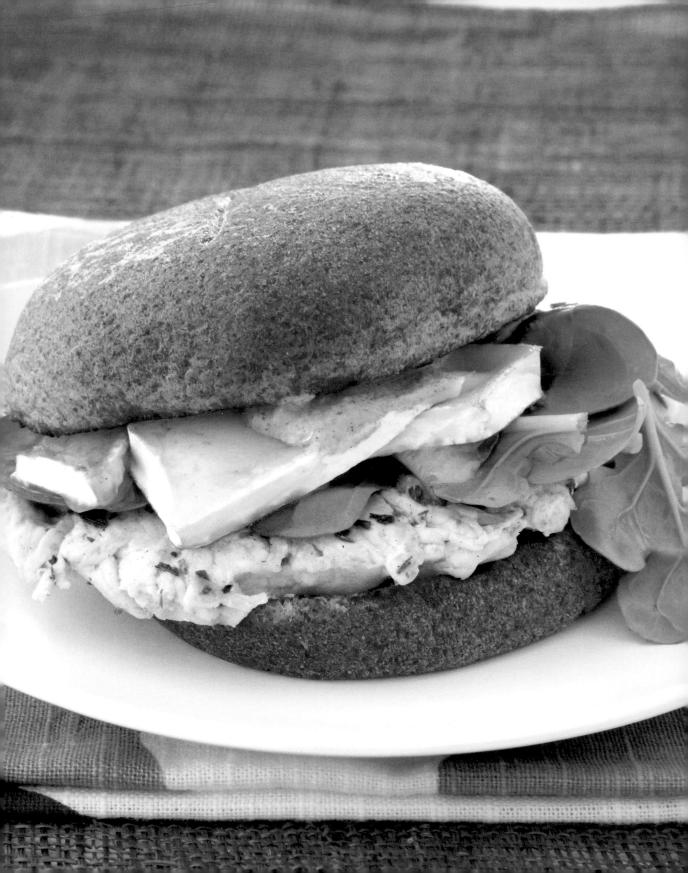

WARM BRIE CHICKEN BREAST SANDWICH

3

I can't count the number of people who have said to me, "My problem is that I love meats and cheeses." And I always reassure them that this isn't actually a problem, even if they're committed to a healthy lifestyle, especially when it comes to meats. I've put in a lot of time over the past twenty years of healthy cooking (and eating!) into resculpting meat dishes, because I do love them myself. Even sausage (see Sweet and Slim Italian Sausage, page 130, and Breakfast Sausage Links, page 44) is no problem these days. Cheese, on the other hand, is a bit tougher. But thanks to a number of companies that offer great lighter cheeses now (trust me, I acknowledge that plenty still offer ones that taste like rubber, or worse), it's not so tough to indulge without consequence.

For this sandwich, I don't peel the Brie. The outer edges have the strongest flavor. So leaving it on means you don't need as much to get that decadent French taste without overindulging. If you prefer the sandwich with the Dijon mustard, it will add about 8 calories, 0 grams of fat, and 98 milligrams of sodium. I like it without because I think the brie flavor is stronger that way, and I'd rather save the extra sodium. If you disagree, feel free to add it.

One 3¹/₂-ounce boneless, skinless chicken breast, visible fat removed
Olive oil spray
¹/₂ teaspoon chopped dried rosemary
Salt and pepper
1 whole-grain hamburger bun
1 ounce light Brie
1¹/₂ teaspoons Dijon mustard, optional
1 small handful arugula leaves

Preheat a grill to high.

Place the chicken breast between two sheets of plastic wrap or wax paper on a flat work surface. Use the flat side of a meat mallet to pound it to an even ¹/₂-inch thickness. Lightly mist the chicken with spray, and then sprinkle it with the rosemary and salt and pepper to taste. Place the chicken on the grill. Turn the heat to medium, if possible, and cook for 3 to 5 minutes per side, until no longer pink inside. During the last minute, place the bun halves, insides facedown, on a top grill rack to toast, watching them carefully. Immediately spread the Brie over the top half of the bun.

Spread the mustard, if using, over the inside of the bun bottom and place it on a plate. Add the chicken breast, then the arugula. Flip the Brie-spread bun atop the sandwich. Serve immediately.

Can be made in 30 minutes or less / No more than 20 minutes hands-on prep time

MAKES 1 SANDWICH; 1 SERVING

3 Each 3-Decadent-Disk serving (1 sandwich) has: 301 calories, 35 g protein, 21 g carbohydrates, 9 g fat, 4 g saturated fat, 73 mg cholesterol, 2 g fiber, 499 mg sodium

HOTTER TURKEY SANDWICH

3

I joke that I was cursed when it comes to food. Though some of my friends say they truly love at least a few veggies, I can't say that I do. (Unless you consider a plate of tomatoes a veggie.) Sure, I eat them, but I don't ever crave them or look forward to them. Add that I love pretty much all meats, bacon, mayonnaise, butter, chocolate, and every variety of cheese known to humankind, and it doesn't exactly set me up to be skinny.

All of that said, I'm actually not a gravy person. It must be the only fattening thing I just couldn't care less about eating. Though I don't crave gravy, I know a lot of other folks do. So to make sure you get your cravings met, I knew I had to include it. This sandwich was the hit of one of my recent taste-testing parties.

1 slice whole-grain bread
4¹/4 ounces Sage Butter Roasted Turkey (page 148), sliced thin, reheated if necessary
2 tablespoons Madeira Wine Gravy (page 149), reheated if necessary

Place the slice of bread on a plate. Top the bread with the turkey and spoon the gravy evenly over the top of the sandwich. Serve immediately.

MAKES 1 SANDWICH; 1 SERVING

 Each 3-Decadent-Disk serving (1 sandwich) has: 294 calories, 38 g protein, 18 g carbohydrates, 6 g fat, 2 g saturated fat, 108 mg cholesterol, 2 g fiber, 541 mg sodium

CURRY CHICKEN WRAP

I'm constantly combining low-fat mayonnaise with other flavors to enrich its taste. The texture is perfect, but when using the low-fat one, I always try to enhance it. For roast beef sandwiches, I'll spike it with a touch of horse-radish. For grilled chicken sandwiches, I might add a bit of chili garlic sauce or chili paste.

Here, I've added curry paste to this creamy chicken salad for a surprisingly easy-to-make pocket reminiscent of Indian cuisine. It's a particularly great recipe for transforming leftover grilled chicken breasts, or you can always purposefully make up a few extras when you are cooking chicken. In a pinch, most grocery stores now sell grilled chicken. Just be sure that you don't buy one with too much sodium, since most curry pastes have more than enough sodium.

4 ounces extra-lean grilled chicken breast or Basic Grilled Chicken (page 61), coarsely chopped
1¹/₂ tablespoons low-fat mayonnaise
1 teaspoon jarred red curry paste
1 (about 8-inch diameter) low-fat, whole-wheat flour tortilla
5 (5-inch-long) cucumber strips, or to taste
5 mango slivers, or to taste
¹/₄ cup red onion slivers

Place the chicken in a medium bowl. Add the mayonnaise and curry paste and stir until well combined.

Place the tortilla on a flat work surface. Lay the cucumber strips in a 3-inch-wide strip down the center, leaving 1 inch bare at one end only. Top with the mango slivers. Spoon the chicken mixture over the mango. Top with the onion. Fold in the bare end, and then roll the sides over to form a burrito-shaped wrap that's open at one end. Serve immediately.

Can be made in 30 minutes or less / No more than 20 minutes hands-on prep time

MAKES 1 WRAP; 1 SERVING

Each 4-Decadent-Disk serving (1 wrap) has: 393 calories, 38 g protein, 40 g carbohydrates, 8 g fat, <1 g saturated fat, 82 mg cholesterol, 4 g fiber, 601 mg sodium

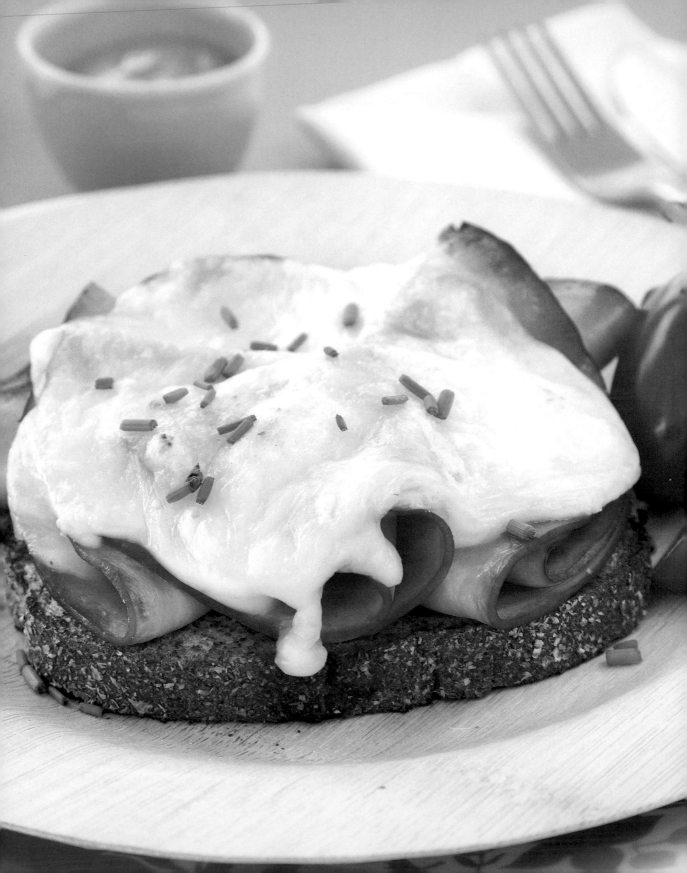

OPEN-FACE HAM AND CHEESE

3

I have very fond early memories of ham. My mom used to cook ham fairly often, then turn it into a kind of ham salad. I remember being so excited to wake up mornings after we'd eaten ham for dinner, because I knew it meant we'd get to put it through the meat grinder. My mom would pull out the meat grinder and sit my sister and me up on the counter. We'd stuff the chunks of ham through the feed tube and it would magically emerge as ground ham. Then we'd add mayonnaise (one of my favorite ingredients at the time) and relish. It was so cool, or was it? What we were thinking eating that?

When I mentioned this sandwich to a friend, he said his family used to have curry cheese sandwiches. They mixed shredded Cheddar with mayo and diced bell peppers, then spread it over a buttered English muffin, sprinkled it with curry powder, and broiled it. Wow! We Americans are great at fattening combos, aren't we? Well, here's a classic combo that seems extra-super-skinny by comparison.

When purchasing the ham for this recipe, be sure to find the one that's lowest in sodium. Also, I've recently been buying 99% lean ham. If you can find that, definitely snag it the next time you're at the grocery store. If you can't, don't

worry. I know it's not so common, so I wrote the recipe for 97% lean knowing that finding the 99% lean one might cause you grief.

1 slice multigrain or seven-grain bread (about 70 calories per slice), lightly toasted
2^1/$_2$ teaspoons honey mustard
3^1/$_2$ ounces shaved 97% fat-free deli ham
One ^{3}/$_4$-ounce slice light Swiss cheese
1 teaspoon minced fresh chives

Preheat the broiler.

Lay the toasted slice of bread on a small nonstick baking sheet. Spread the mustard evenly over the slice. Then top evenly with the ham, followed by the cheese. Place the sheet on the top oven rack and broil for 1 to 2 minutes, or until the cheese is melted and the ham is warmed through.

Transfer the sandwich to a plate and sprinkle with chives. Serve immediately.

Can be made in 30 minutes or less / No more than 20 minutes hands-on prep time

MAKES 1 SANDWICH; 1 SERVING

3 Each 3-Decadent-Disk serving (1 sandwich) has: 290 calories, 29 g protein, 28 g carbohydrates, 7 g fat, 2 g saturated fat, 57 mg cholesterol, 2 g fiber, 1,289 mg sodium

You save: 150 calories, 21 g fat, 14 g saturated fat

Traditional serving: 440 calories, 23 g protein, 26 g carbohydrates, 28 g fat, 16 g saturated fat, 95 mg cholesterol, fiber N/A, 1,401 mg sodium

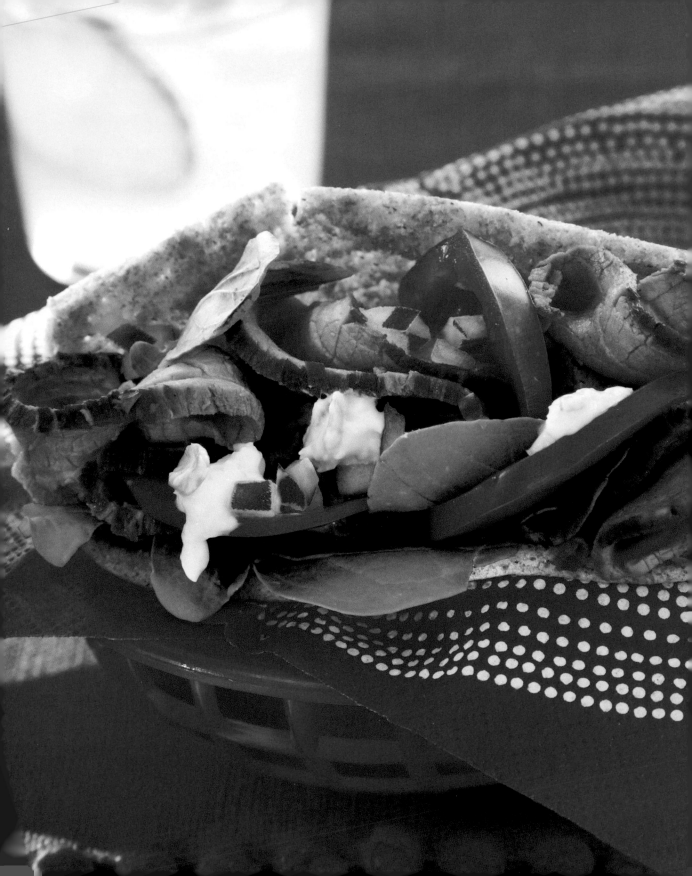

GOURMET ROAST BEEF POCKET

This sandwich is a great example of how quick it can be to bang out a tasty meal. If you've made Roast Beef with Horseradish Cream for dinner, it takes seconds to throw this together. If you haven't, you can always substitute extra-lean roast beef from your local deli and do a quick mixture of low-fat mayonnaise and horseradish instead of the horseradish cream. Either way, you can have it wrapped up and be out the door in five minutes.

1 (about 6^1/$_2$-inch diameter) whole-wheat pita circle
1^1/$_2$ tablespoons Horseradish Cream (page 122)
^{1}/$_2$ cup arugula leaves
2 tablespoons chopped red onion
3^1/$_2$ ounces thinly sliced Roast Beef (page 121), or extra-lean shaved deli roast beef
Three ^{1}/$_4$-inch-thick tomato slices

Place the pita on a cutting board. Cut off a third of the pita circle and save that piece for another use, such as for dipping with Mediterranean Layer Dip (page 197) or Bacon Horseradish Dip (page 205). Spread the Horseradish Cream evenly on one side of the inside of the pocket. Add the arugula and onion, then the roast beef and tomato slices. Serve immediately, or wrap in plastic wrap and refrigerate for up to 8 hours.

Can be made in 30 minutes or less / No more than 20 minutes hands-on prep time

MAKES 1 POCKET; 1 SERVING

Each 3-Decadent-Disk serving (1 pocket) has: 300 calories, 33 g protein, 26 g carbohydrates, 7 g fat, 3 g saturated fat, 61 mg cholesterol, 4 g fiber, 393 mg sodium

OPEN-ENDED BUFFALO CHICKEN WRAP

I started making open-ended wraps years ago when I realized how much tortilla it took to cover a standard-sized serving (4 ounces) of lean protein plus the veggies you want to add to your meals any time you can. So instead of using the burrito-sized tortillas, which often have 160 to 200 calories and 5 to 10 grams of fat, I stick to the low-fat, 8-inch ones with only 110 to 120 calories and 2 grams of fat. Then I just stuff them with chicken, turkey, or other lean protein followed by some onions, bell pepper strips, or other veggies and leave part of the filling uncovered. In this case, the creaminess of the coleslaw coupled with the spicy buffalo strips make the perfect pick-up-able package.

1 (about 8-inch diameter) low-fat, whole-wheat flour tortilla
$^1/_2$ cup Colorful Coleslaw (page 189)
4 Boneless Buffalo Strips (page 195)
Hot sauce (a thick one, like Frank's; see page 17)

Place the tortilla on a flat work surface. Spread the Colorful Coleslaw in a 3-inch-wide strip down the center, leaving about 1 inch bare at one end only. Place the Boneless Buffalo Strips over the coleslaw. Drizzle hot sauce to taste over the strips. Fold in the bare end, and then roll the sides over to form a burrito-shaped wrap that's open at one end. Serve immediately.

MAKES 1 WRAP; 1 SERVING

 Each 3-Decadent-Disk serving (1 wrap) has: 293 calories, 25 g protein, 34 g carbohydrates, 8 g fat, 2 g saturated fat, 58 mg cholesterol, 4 g fiber, 621 mg sodium

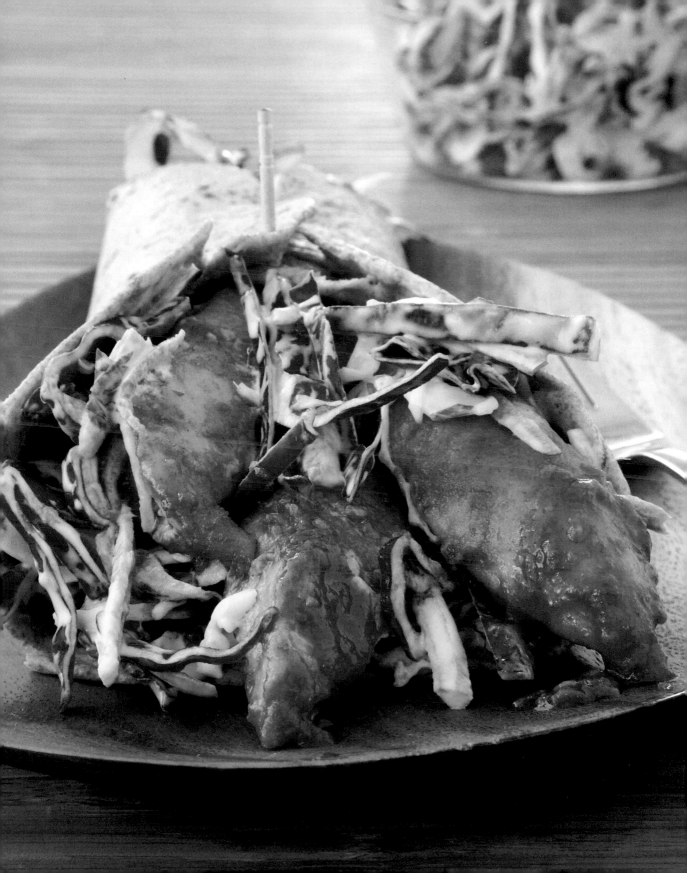

RENOVATED REUBEN WRAP

3

I was recently at a New York City deli with my friend Jim. It was the night before I was being photographed for the cover of this book, so I didn't want to eat anything too heavy or full of sodium. I ordered a simple, lean roast beef sandwich, planning to eat half, since I know they pack them so full.

So Jim and I were sitting catching up when a waiter plopped down a huge mound of food at a nearby table. By "mound," I mean at least 1^1/2 to 2 pounds of corned beef, tons of cheese, Russian dressing, rye bread, and so on, and it was served to one woman. I was shocked by the portion size.

I debated cutting this recipe when I realized how much sodium was in it and that I couldn't find a brand of corned beef that didn't have quite a bit. But then when I realized how much is in a typical Reuben, I figured this is definitely, by far, the lesser of two evils. Just please don't make this a staple in your diet. It has more sodium than any other recipe in this book. It's great for an occasional craving, but definitely not every day. Also, make sure to drain the sauerkraut before putting it in the sandwich. It should be measured after being drained through a sieve to release excess moisture, not before.

1^1/2 tablespoons Russian Dressing (recipe follows)
1 (about 8-inch diameter) low-fat, whole-wheat flour tortilla
1 ounce (^{1}/2 cup) finely shredded light Swiss cheese
3 ounces 98% fat-free deli-style corned beef
^{1}/4 cup well-drained, refrigerated sauerkraut

Prepare the Russian Dressing.

Preheat a medium nonstick skillet over medium heat. Lay the tortilla flat in the pan. After 30 seconds, flip it. Then sprinkle the cheese in an even strip (about 3 inches wide) down the center of the tortilla, leaving about 2 inches bare on one end. Cover the pan just long enough to melt the cheese and heat the tortilla, 1 to 2 minutes. Remove the lid and top the cheese evenly with the corned beef, then the sauerkraut and the dressing. Transfer the tortilla with filling to a flat work surface. Fold in the bare end, and then roll the sides over to form a burrito-shaped wrap that's open at one end. Serve immediately.   *(continued)*

Can be made in 30 minutes or less / No more than 20 minutes hands-on prep time

MAKES 1 WRAP; 1 SERVING

3 Each 3-Decadent-Disk serving (1 wrap) has: 309 calories, 27 g protein, 29 g carbohydrates, 9 g fat, 4 g saturated fat, 55 mg cholesterol, 3 g fiber, 1,300 mg sodium
You save: 215 calories, 23 g fat, 10 g saturated fat
Traditional serving: 524 calories, 26 g protein, 34 g carbohydrates, 32 g fat, 14 g saturated fat, 92 mg cholesterol, 3 g fiber, 1,587 mg sodium

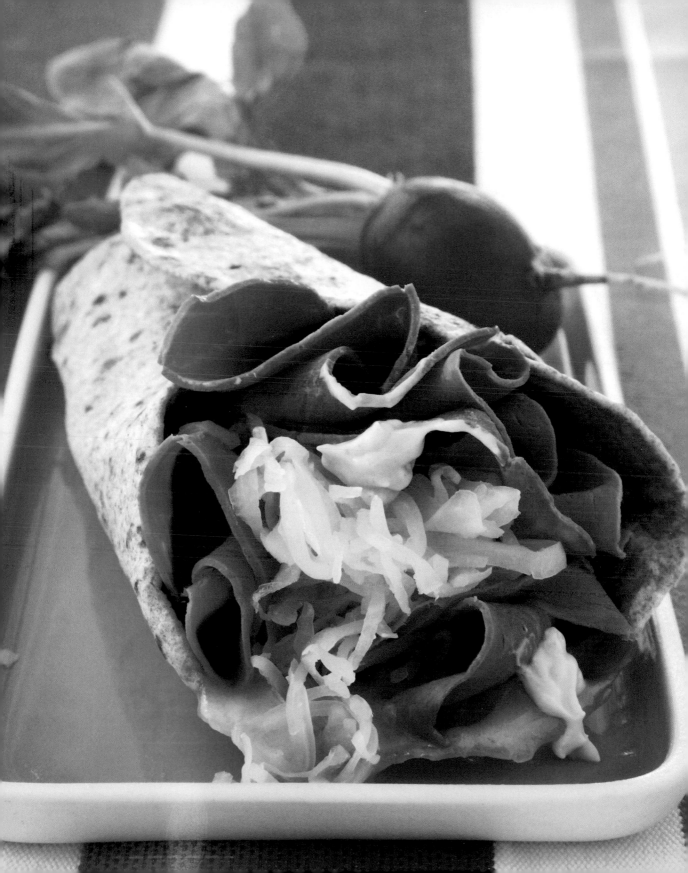

I found lots of different Reuben sandwich recipes, ranging anywhere from 1,500 milligrams of sodium to more than 4,000 milligrams for the big, deli-style sandwiches stacked with piles of corned beef. Even if you compare my homemade version of the sandwich (which is not as insanely thick as one you might see at a deli) to a similar homemade version, you'll still save nearly 20 percent of the sodium by making the *Most Decadent Diet Ever!* version.

RUSSIAN DRESSING

3 tablespoons low-fat mayonnaise
1^1/$_2$ tablespoons ketchup
1 tablespoon minced onion
^{1}/$_4$ teaspoon bottled horseradish
^{1}/$_4$ teaspoon Worcestershire sauce

Mix all of the ingredients in a small bowl until well combined.

Makes 5^1/$_2$ tablespoons
Each tablespoon has: 19 calories, trace protein, 2 g carbohydrates, 1 g fat, 0 g saturated fat, trace cholesterol, trace fiber, 49 mg sodium

MOST PEOPLE THINK OF SALADS AS diet food. But are they always? They can be some of the greatest evils to a healthy eater, because they are often shockingly full of fat and calories. So often restaurant salads with all of their cheese, fried noodles, rich salad dressing, and so on, have more than 1,000 calories and 75 grams of fat. Granted, that is for a larger-sized serving than we should be eating.

For years, I ate salads when I went out, thinking I was being "good." How I thought ordering a Caesar salad wouldn't set me back is beyond me. Sometimes I still order them, thinking I'm doing myself a favor. I just can't seem to wrap my brain around the notion that they are, by far, the "worst" thing I eat. I think it's in part because I really believed for so many years they were great for me.

But in the last few years, as I've been doing so many makeovers of restaurant favorites, I've been shocked to learn that salads not only are some of the highest-fat items on menus, they're some of the hardest to make over in a lean way.

Look at this chapter. The decadent salads included here are awesome and, in many cases, higher in fat than most of the other dishes in the book. So if you're really, truly a salad lover, go crazy in this chapter. If you have other ways to get your veggies that you enjoy as much while noshing on your burgers, that's probably a better strategy for you.

All of this negative talk about salads isn't the whole story. Salads can actually be saviors. I was recently in my friend Michelle's wedding and had to drive to Modesto, which was a good seven hours from Los Angeles in Memorial Day weekend traffic. I knew I didn't want to rely on rest stops, so I packed a few salads for the weekend and stuck them in the cooler in my car. They now have these great coolers that plug into your car and also have an adapter to plug into your office or hotel room. They're the best for setting yourself up to eat healthy on road trips whether you're packing your favorite salad or a sandwich or two.

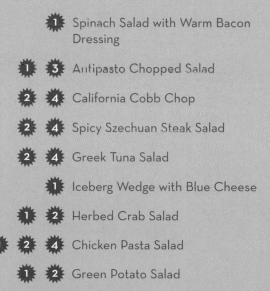

1 Spinach Salad with Warm Bacon Dressing

1 3 Antipasto Chopped Salad

2 4 California Cobb Chop

2 4 Spicy Szechuan Steak Salad

2 4 Greek Tuna Salad

1 Iceberg Wedge with Blue Cheese

1 2 Herbed Crab Salad

1 2 4 Chicken Pasta Salad

1 2 Green Potato Salad

SPINACH SALAD WITH WARM BACON DRESSING

I find it fascinating that I can make a Chocolate Not-Only-in-Your-Dreams Cake (page 210) and other rich, decadent, insanely chocolaty desserts with only 1 or 2 grams of fat, but can rarely make over an entrée-sized salad for less than 10. Oddly, this is one case where even though this recipe sounds insanely fattening, I can.

A large serving of this salad has so few fat grams and calories it shocks me, so I eat it often. And so I never get tired of it, I often add grilled chicken, egg whites, shrimp, and/or red onion. You can add 3¹/₂ ounces of grilled shrimp or chicken (see Basic Grilled Chicken, page 61) for only about another 100 calories, or a hard-boiled egg white for only 17 calories, and turn it into a great entrée. Or add a few dried tart cherries or a touch of reduced-fat blue cheese to make it extra-special. To take it to lunch, simply pack the dressing separately and reheat it in the microwave at work just before tossing and eating. You'll be the envy of your co-workers.

3 cups loosely packed baby spinach leaves
¹/₂ cup sliced button mushrooms
2 tablespoons Warm Bacon Dressing (recipe follows), reheated if necessary

Combine the spinach and mushrooms in a medium bowl. Add the Warm Bacon Dressing and toss until combined. Serve immediately.

WARM BACON DRESSING

1 tablespoon Dijon mustard
1¹/₂ tablespoons honey
2 teaspoons unbleached all-purpose flour
¹/₄ cup fat-free, lower-sodium chicken broth
2 tablespoons cider vinegar
3 slices center-cut bacon, finely chopped
1 garlic clove, minced
2 tablespoons minced shallots
Black pepper

Whisk the mustard, honey, and flour in a small mixing bowl. When smooth, slowly whisk in the chicken broth, then the vinegar.

Place a small nonstick saucepan over medium-high heat. Put in the bacon and cook, stirring frequently, until crisp, 4 to 6 minutes. Stir in the garlic and shallots and reduce the heat to medium. Cook for about 30 seconds, or until fragrant. Whisk in the mustard mixture and reduce until thickened slightly, stirring frequently, 1 to 2 minutes. Season with pepper to taste. The dressing can be made up to 5 days in advance and refrigerated in an airtight container, then reheated before use.

Makes about 9 tablespoons
Each tablespoon has: 35 calories, <1 g protein, 4 g carbohydrates, 2 g fat, <1 g saturated fat, 4 mg cholesterol, trace fiber, 79 mg sodium

---

Can be made in 30 minutes or less / No more than 20 minutes hands-on prep time

MAKES 1 SALAD; 1 SERVING

 Each 1-Decadent-Disk serving (1 salad) has: 108 calories, 4 g protein, 16 g carbohydrates, 4 g fat, 2 g saturated fat, 7 mg cholesterol, 4 g fiber, 275 mg sodium

ANTIPASTO CHOPPED SALAD

🌟 🌟

I am a huge fan of chopped salads. When veggies are chopped finely, you get a flavor explosion in your mouth as the ingredients mingle, thus requiring significantly less dressing. There are two key things to remember when attempting to master the perfect, restaurant-quality salad—always dry the lettuce well and remove the seeds from tomatoes and cucumbers. If you omit either of these steps, you're pretty much guaranteeing a soggy salad.

Feel free to add freshly minced garlic, crushed red pepper flakes, or more chiles to this salad if you like a little more kick. They'll add negligible amounts of fat and calories and just might get you completely addicted to eating this tasty fare over much fattier options. Also, if it's available in your area, use 99% lean ham. The 97% lean ham has about 122 calories and 2 grams of fat per 4-ounce serving; the 99% lean variety has only 100 calories and 1 gram of fat per 4-ounce serving. I've found it equally delicious and would recommend using the 99% lean version in all recipes that call for sliced deli ham.

3 cups finely shredded romaine lettuce

2 cups finely shredded arugula leaves

$^1/_4$ cup finely slivered fresh basil leaves (see page 20)

$1^1/_4$ ounces (about $^1/_3$ cup) shredded low-fat mozzarella ($2^1/_2$ grams of fat or less per ounce), divided

1 ounce (about $^1/_4$ cup) $^1/_4$-inch cubes 97% lean deli ham

1 ounce (about $^1/_4$ cup) slivers or $^1/_4$-inch cubes reduced-fat salami

1 medium Roma tomato, seeded and finely chopped (about $^1/_2$ cup; see page 21)

$^1/_4$ cup finely slivered roasted red bell pepper (see page 20)

$^1/_2$ teaspoon minced jarred hot chiles, or more to taste

2 tablespoons Red Wine Vinaigrette (recipe follows)

Combine the lettuce, arugula, basil, mozzarella, ham, salami, tomato, bell pepper, and chiles in a large bowl and toss until well combined. Add the Red Wine Vinaigrette and toss until the dressing is evenly distributed. Serve immediately. *(continued)*

Can be made in 30 minutes or less

MAKES 5 CUPS; 1 (ENTRÉE) SERVING OR 3 (APPETIZER) PORTIONS

🌟 Each 1-Decadent-Disk portion (about $1^2/_3$ cups) has: 101 calories, 8 g protein, 7 g carbohydrates, 5 g fat, 1 g saturated fat, 13 mg cholesterol, 3 g fiber, 306 mg sodium

🌟 Each 3-Decadent-Disk serving (5 cups) has: 304 calories, 23 g protein, 22 g carbohydrates, 16 g fat, 4 g saturated fat, 38 mg cholesterol, 8 g fiber, 919 mg sodium

RED WINE VINAIGRETTE

2 tablespoons red wine vinegar
1¹/₂ tablespoons honey mustard
¹/₂ teaspoon honey
1 teaspoon minced fresh garlic
1 tablespoon extra virgin olive oil
Pinch of salt
Black pepper

Whisk the vinegar, mustard, honey, and garlic in a small bowl. Slowly whisk in the olive oil. Season with salt and pepper to taste. The dressing can be made up to 5 days in advance and stored in the refrigerator.

Makes a bit more than 4 tablespoons
Each 2-tablespoon serving has: 91 calories, <1 g protein, 6 g carbohydrates, 8 g fat, 1 g saturated fat, trace cholesterol, <1 g fiber, 132 mg sodium

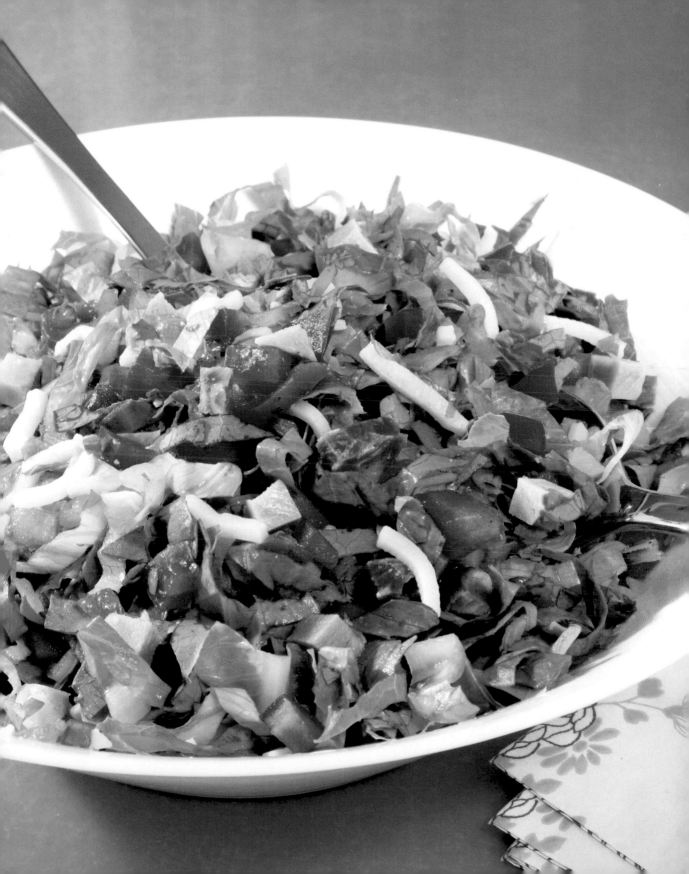

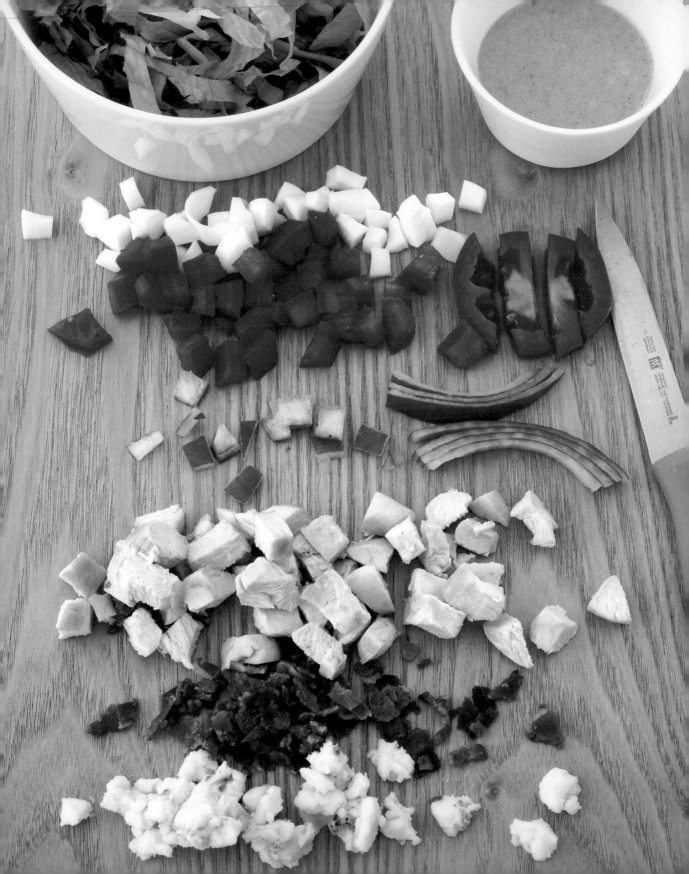

CALIFORNIA COBB CHOP

2 4

Though iceberg lettuce is seemingly the most commonly eaten lettuce in most parts of the country, it doesn't have as many nutrients as darker varieties of lettuce. I always try to add darker lettuces to my salads and sandwiches when I can (though sometimes you just need that crunch of a romaine or iceberg). In the Antipasto Chopped Salad (page 85) I add arugula. Here, I add spinach. In the case of the Antipasto Chopped Salad, I didn't want to use all arugula because it has such a strong flavor; I didn't want it to overpower the other ingredients. If I were to make this one with all spinach, the spinach might seem a bit soggy. But by using a little less than half, I'm getting the crunch of the iceberg with some of the nutrients and added fiber of the spinach.

To save time, feel free to use a low-fat, store-bought salad dressing if you've found a brand you love. Though I do like a few brands, many just don't meet my personal decadence requirement.

2 slices center-cut bacon

2 cups finely shredded romaine lettuce

1¹/₂ cups finely shredded spinach leaves

4 ounces finely chopped grilled chicken breast, Basic Grilled Chicken (page 61), or extra-lean roasted turkey

³/₄ cup seeded and finely chopped tomatoes (see page 21)

1 large hard-boiled egg white, finely chopped

¹/₂ ounce (about 2 tablespoons) crumbled reduced-fat blue cheese

2 tablespoons finely chopped red onion

2 tablespoons Red Wine Vinaigrette (page 86)

Place a small nonstick skillet over medium heat. Put in the bacon strips, side by side, and cook for 6 to 8 minutes, flipping every couple of minutes, until crispy and well done. Transfer the bacon to a paper towel–lined plate to drain and cool. After the slices are cooled, finely chop them.

Combine the bacon, lettuce, spinach, chicken, tomatoes, egg white, cheese, and onion in a large bowl. Add the Red Wine Vinaigrette and toss until well combined. Serve immediately.

MAKES 5 CUPS; 1 (ENTRÉE) SERVING OR 2 (APPETIZER) PORTIONS

2 Each 2-Decadent-Disk portion (2¹/₂ cups) has: 195 calories, 21 g protein, 10 g carbohydrates, 9 g fat, 3 g saturated fat, 43 mg cholesterol, 3 g fiber, 394 mg sodium

4 Each 4-Decadent-Disk serving (5 cups) has: 390 calories, 41 g protein, 19 g carbohydrates, 17 g fat, 5 g saturated fat, 87 mg cholesterol, 6 g fiber, 752 mg sodium

You save: 158 calories, 26 g fat, 6 g saturated fat

Traditional serving: 548 calories, 32 g protein, 9 g carbohydrates, 43 g fat, 11 g saturated fat, 193 mg cholesterol, fiber N/A, 898 mg sodium

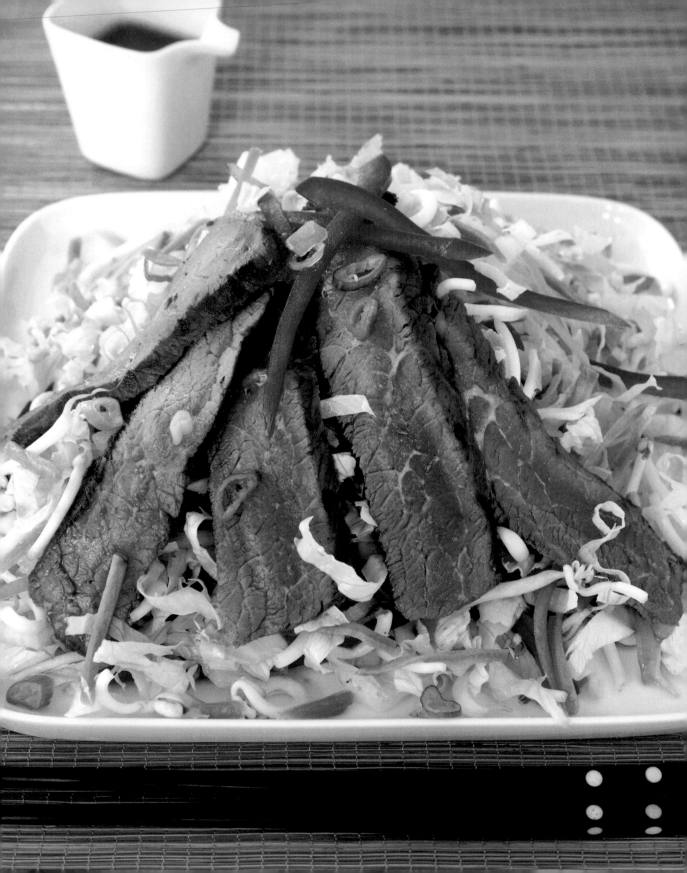

SPICY SZECHUAN STEAK SALAD

I would prefer eating a salad over a hot veggie any day. And I've always been like that. I've spent a lot of time over the years re-creating every salad I've really enjoyed in restaurants. Here is a take on one that I ate frequently until I realized just how much fat and how many calories the original contained. Now I can make it on my own and enjoy it with much less guilt.

This salad is especially great because the dressing lasts a long time. You can make it and then throw the salad together in minutes. Also, to save time, you can use any extra-lean grilled steak (it's best to stick to a variety seasoned with just olive oil, salt, and pepper or one with an Asian flair). The dressing is very flavorful, so you don't need the Szechuan seasoning to enjoy it.

4 cups finely shredded romaine lettuce
$^1/_2$ cup finely slivered red bell pepper (see page 20)
$^1/_2$ cup finely slivered carrot (see page 20)
$^1/_2$ cup slivered Chinese snow peas
$^1/_2$ cup mung bean sprouts
3 tablespoons Szechuan Dressing (recipe follows)
$^1/_4$ cup chopped whole green onions
4$^3/_4$ ounces Spicy Szechuan Steak (page 114), sliced into thin strips

Combine the lettuce, bell pepper, carrot, peas, and sprouts in a large bowl. Add the Szechuan Dressing and toss. Sprinkle the onions over the top. Top with the steak strips. Serve immediately.

SZECHUAN DRESSING

2 tablespoons rice wine vinegar
2 tablespoons Szechuan sauce
2 tablespoons honey
1 teaspoon prepared hot mustard
2 teaspoons extra virgin olive oil
1 teaspoon toasted sesame oil

Whisk together the vinegar, Szechuan sauce, honey, and mustard in a small resealable container. Gradually whisk in the oils. Serve immediately or refrigerate for up to 5 days.

Makes about 1/2 cup
Each 2-tablespoon serving has: 77 calories, trace protein, 11 g carbohydrates, 4 g fat, <1 g saturated fat, trace cholesterol, trace fiber, 66 mg sodium

---

Can be made in 30 minutes or less

MAKES 1 SALAD; 1 (ENTRÉE) SERVING OR 2 (APPETIZER) PORTIONS

 Each 2-Decadent-Disk portion ($^1/_2$ salad) has: 195 calories, 17 g protein, 23 g carbohydrates, 6 g fat, 1 g saturated fat, 28 mg cholesterol, 6 g fiber, 153 mg sodium

Each 4-Decadent-Disk serving (1 salad) has: 390 calories, 34 g protein, 45 g carbohydrates, 12 g fat, 3 g saturated fat, 56 mg cholesterol, 11 g fiber, 305 mg sodium

You save: 39 calories, 15 g fat, 4 g saturated fat

Traditional serving: 429 calories, 34 g protein, 13 g carbohydrates, 27 g fat, 7 g saturated fat, 71 mg cholesterol, 6 g fiber, 419 mg sodium

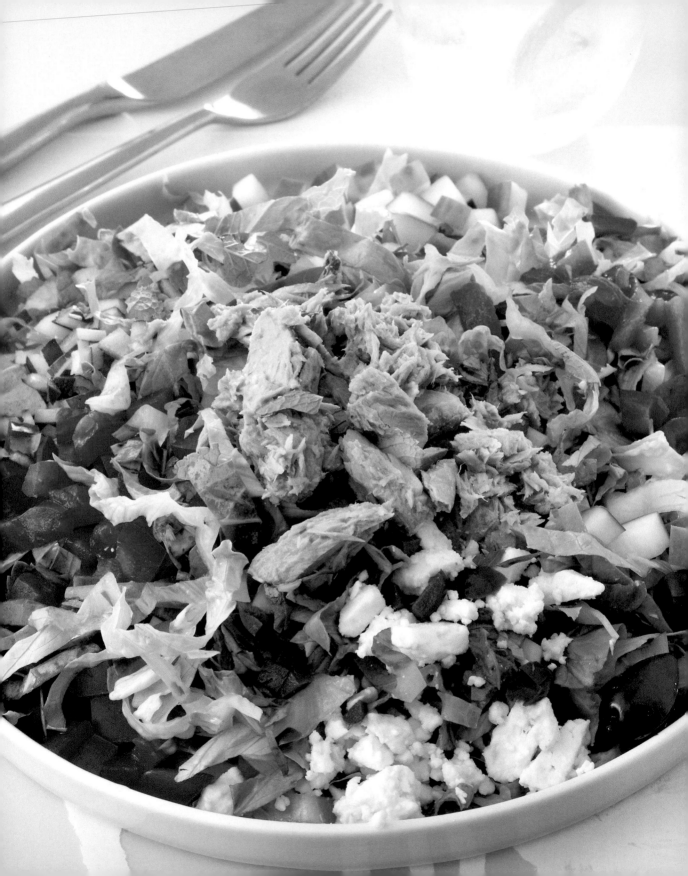

GREEK TUNA SALAD

My friend Alana recently took me to a French bistro just outside Beverly Hills for lunch. They had the best Greek tuna salad. I'd never paired canned tuna with Greek ingredients, but I loved it. This version tastes very similar to the one I had at the restaurant. But I'll be honest: when I haven't been eating much sodium or fat or I've done an exceptionally great workout, I spike it with a few more olives and a bit more feta. It's great the way it is, but it's beyond amazing with the extras. What I find fascinating is that this is already on the higher side in terms of fat content as compared to other dishes in this book, even using reduced-fat ingredients and much-lower-fat dressing. It really makes you wonder about traditional Greek salads.

Note that if you don't mind it, it's best to use lower-sodium tuna. This dish is exceptionally high in sodium as is (though it would be much higher in a restaurant). Also, if you find a brand you like, you can always save more fat by using fat-free feta. You'll save an additional 16 calories and 2 grams of fat in this salad.

2 tablespoons fresh lemon juice (about 1 lemon), or more to taste

2 teaspoons extra virgin olive oil

4 Kalamata olives, finely chopped, or more to taste

1 teaspoon minced fresh garlic (about 1 small clove)

3 cups finely shredded romaine lettuce

1/2 cup seeded and finely chopped tomato (about 1 medium tomato; see page 21)

1/3 cup roasted red bell pepper strips (see page 20)

1/4 cup seeded and finely chopped cucumber (see page 21)

3 tablespoons finely chopped red onion

2 tablespoons finely chopped fresh mint

2 tablespoons finely chopped fresh flat-leaf parsley

3/4 ounce (about 3 tablespoons) reduced-fat feta cheese, crumbled, or more to taste

4 1/2 ounces drained canned or pouch chunk light tuna

Whisk the lemon juice and olive oil in a small bowl. Stir in the olives and garlic.

Combine the lettuce, tomato, bell pepper, cucumber, onion, mint, parsley, 2 tablespoons feta, and half of the tuna in a large bowl. Pour the lemon juice mixture over the top and toss until well combined. Mound the remaining tuna on top, and then top that with the remaining feta. Serve immediately.

Can be made in 30 minutes or less

MAKES 1 SALAD; 1 (ENTRÉE) SERVING OR 2 (APPETIZER) PORTIONS

2 Each 2-Decadent-Disk portion (1/2 salad) has: 200 calories, 22 g protein, 12 g carbohydrates, 7 g fat, 2 g saturated fat, 43 mg cholesterol, 4 g fiber, 544 mg sodium

4 Each 4-Decadent-Disk serving (1 salad) has: 400 calories, 43 g protein, 24 g carbohydrates, 15 g fat, 4 g saturated fat, 86 mg cholesterol, 8 g fiber, 1,088 mg sodium

ICEBERG WEDGE WITH BLUE CHEESE

For years nutritionists have told us that we should eat darker greens instead of iceberg lettuce because they have more nutrients. In finer restaurants you almost always see mixed greens, especially the popular mesclun mix. Spinach salads are very popular, too, and many people trying to eat healthier order them for all of their health benefits. But go to your local steakhouse and you're likely to be enticed by the iceberg wedge slathered in blue cheese. And now it's starting to appear on other menus in my area. That scares me, given the obesity epidemic we're facing. It is, in essence, a big pile of water with a huge amount of fat slathered on top. True, most restaurants serve it with at least a few tomatoes, which do have antioxidants. But seriously, be careful. A typical creamy salad dressing has about 180 calories and 18 to 20 grams of fat for 2 tablespoons. Those little to-go salad dressing cups tend to look tiny, yet house $1/4$ cup. That's 4 tablespoons. And most often, you walk out the door with two of them. So that means, if you're actually eating it all, you're consuming about 720 calories and 72 to 80 grams of fat in the salad dressing alone. Really makes you think, doesn't it?

1 small head iceberg lettuce
$3/4$ cup Blue Cheese Dressing (page 196), divided
1 medium Roma tomato, seeded and finely chopped (about $1/2$ cup; see page 21), divided
2 tablespoons finely chopped whole green onion, divided
Salt and pepper

Hold the head of lettuce, core facedown, over a clean work surface and slam it down to release the core. Grab the core and pull it out to remove it. Hold the head of lettuce under cold running water, rotating it to rinse it well. Shake it to remove excess water, then allow it to dry on paper towels. It should be thoroughly dry. Peel off any outer leaves that look wilted. Then place the head on a cutting board, open side down. Cut the head into 4 wedges.

Place each wedge on a salad plate and spoon 3 tablespoons Blue Cheese Dressing over each. Then sprinkle a quarter of the tomato and a quarter of the onion evenly over each wedge. Season with salt and pepper to taste. Serve immediately.

Can be made in 30 minutes or less / No more than 20 minutes hands-on prep time

MAKES 4 WEDGES, 4 SERVINGS

Each 1-Decadent-Disk serving (1 wedge) has: 110 calories, 5 g protein, 7 g carbohydrates, 7 g fat, 2 g saturated fat, 12 mg cholesterol, 2 g fiber, 320 mg sodium

You save: 100 calories, 12 g fat, 3 g saturated fat

Traditional serving: 210 calories, 5 g protein, 6 g carbohydrates, 19 g fat, 5 g saturated fat, 14 mg cholesterol, 1 g fiber, 503 mg sodium

HERBED CRAB SALAD

🟊1 🟊2

I grew up in Wyomissing, Pennsylvania, where there was a local farmers' market that was open only on Thursdays and Fridays. Every Friday afternoon, my mom rushed out to "make it to the farmers' market." She often took my sister and me with her, and we always had our assignments. I picked up the crab salad and roasted-in-the-shell peanuts for my dad. Leslie usually went to the lunchmeat counter, and my mom grabbed all of the fruits and veggies.

As I got older and realized just how fattening that crab salad was that my dad was still eating (and loved!), I developed this one, which is very similar, to replace it. It's one of my assistant Lindsey's favorite dishes in the book. You'd be surprised how many times we "tested" it simply to satisfy her craving.

¼ cup plus 1 tablespoon light mayonnaise
2 tablespoons fat-free milk
2 tablespoons fat-free plain yogurt
1 pound imitation crabmeat, coarsely shredded
2 tablespoons finely chopped whole green onion
2 tablespoons finely chopped red onion
2 tablespoons finely chopped fresh dill
2 tablespoons chopped fresh parsley

Whisk the mayonnaise, milk, and yogurt in a large resealable plastic container until well combined and smooth. Add the crabmeat, green onion, red onion, dill, and parsley. Stir until well combined. Seal the container and refrigerate for at least 6 hours, or overnight for optimum flavor.

The *Most Decadent Diet Ever!* version is even bigger than the one I've compared it to, yet it's significantly less fat and calories.

Can be made in 30 minutes or less

MAKES ABOUT 3½ CUPS; 4 SERVINGS OR 8 PORTIONS

🟊1 Each 1-Decadent-Disk portion (heaping ⅓ cup) has: 99 calories, 8 g protein, 9 g carbohydrates, 3 g fat, trace saturated fat, 30 mg cholesterol, trace fiber, 115 mg sodium

🟊2 Each 2-Decadent-Disk serving (heaping ¾ cup) has: 198 calories, 16 g protein, 17 g carbohydrates, 6 fat, <1 g saturated fat, 61 mg cholesterol, <1 g fiber, 230 mg sodium

You save: 372 calories, 47 g fat, 27 g saturated fat

Traditional serving: 570 calories, 11 g protein, 13 g carbohydrates, 53 g fat, 27 g saturated fat, 72 mg cholesterol, trace fiber, 1,108 mg sodium

CHICKEN PASTA SALAD

1 2 4

This dish was probably one of the most frustrating in the book to get right—in part, because it is so difficult to make a quality pasta salad without tons of oil, and people just don't realize that until they make one on their own.

Before I owned a catering business, I worked for others. At one, we made a Greek pasta salad that was out of this world. The bad thing, however, was the insane amount of olive oil used. We'd make it the day before a job and the oil would soak in. When we'd get to the job, we'd add another cup or so to make it glisten and look ultra-fresh again. That would also soak in within hours. So we'd add even more. But the salad tasted as though it was only lightly coated. In actuality a small serving could have up to 300 calories and close to 35 grams of fat.

After testing a creamy version of this salad, then a pesto version, neither of which was exciting me, I arrived at this one. By adding tons of fresh raw veggies, I didn't need as much dressing and I ended up with a bigger portion than normal for so few calories. I love lots of red wine vinegar. If you're not as much of a fan, just add a touch. If you're like me, feel free to go crazy without consequence. Vinegar has only 11 calories and no fat per $1/4$ cup.

$3/4$ pound Basic Grilled Chicken (page 61) or other lean grilled chicken, cut into 2-inch strips
1 recipe Red Wine Vinaigrette (page 86)
8 ounces dried penne pasta
$3/4$ cup matchstick-sized red bell pepper strips (see page 20)
$3/4$ cup matchstick-sized green bell pepper strips (see page 20)
$1/2$ cup sun-dried tomatoes, cut into matchstick-sized pieces
$1/2$ cup red onion slivers
$2^1/2$ tablespoons canned chopped black olives
1 tablespoon minced fresh garlic
$1^1/2$ teaspoons finely chopped fresh oregano
Red wine vinegar
Black pepper

Prepare the chicken if necessary.

Prepare the Red Wine Vinaigrette.

Cook the pasta according to package directions. Drain it and run under cold water. Shake off any excess water.

Combine the chicken, pasta, bell peppers, tomatoes, onion, olives, garlic, and oregano in a large bowl. Add the dressing and toss until well combined. Season with red wine vinegar and black pepper to taste. Serve immediately.

MAKES 10$1/2$ TO 11 CUPS; 4 SERVINGS OR 8 OR 16 PORTIONS

1 Each 1-Decadent-Disk portion (about $2/3$ cup) has: 101 calories, 7 g protein, 14 g carbohydrates, 2 g fat, <1 g saturated fat, 12 mg cholesterol, 1 g fiber, 87 mg sodium

2 Each 2-Decadent-Disk portion (about $1^1/4$ cups) has: 203 calories, 15 g protein, 28 g carbohydrates, 4 g fat, 1 g saturated fat, 24 mg cholesterol, 2 g fiber, 174 mg sodium

4 Each 4-Decadent-Disk serving (about $2^1/2$ cups) has: 406 calories, 29 g protein, 55 g carbohydrates, 8 g fat, 1 g saturated fat, 49 mg cholesterol, 4 g fiber, 349 mg sodium

You save: 190 calories, 31 g fat, 5 g saturated fat

Traditional serving: 596 calories, 22 g protein, 43 g carbohydrates, 39 g fat, 6 g saturated fat, 36 mg cholesterol, 5 g fiber, 856 mg sodium

GREEN POTATO SALAD

1 **2**

I went on a handful of dates with a guy who was the CFO of an herb company. He told me that his company sold more basil and mint than any other herbs. Basil apparently used to win by an even greater margin, but with the strong emergence of the mojito lately, mint sales have seriously skyrocketed. He brought me big boxes of herbs every week. Because they add so much flavor and are virtually calorie free, I always use a lot, but I started making a point of creating dishes from them while I had access in bulk for free. This is one of my favorites.

When you're making this potato salad, I highly recommend that you mash the potatoes a bit as you stir them. It gives the salad a creamier texture, eliminating the need for a lot of mayonnaise or dressing. Larger chunks of potatoes will seem drier. Also note that potatoes are one of those foods that definitely require adding salt. Be sure to season this one well to taste.

$2^1/4$ pounds baking potatoes, peeled and cut into
   1-inch pieces
Salt
$3/4$ cup fat-free plain yogurt
2 teaspoons Dijon mustard
1 tablespoon plus 1 teaspoon extra virgin olive oil
$2/3$ cup finely chopped whole green onions
3 tablespoons finely chopped fresh parsley
2 tablespoons finely chopped fresh dill
Black pepper

Cook the potatoes in a pot of boiling salted water until tender, 12 to 15 minutes. Drain and cool to room temperature.

Meanwhile, whisk the yogurt and mustard in a small bowl. Slowly whisk in the olive oil. Add the onions, parsley, and dill and stir until combined.

Transfer the potatoes to a large bowl and pour the yogurt mixture over them. Mix well with a wooden spoon, breaking some of the potatoes, so that some of them are a bit mashed and the ingredients are well combined. Season generously with salt and pepper to taste. Refrigerate for 1 hour to 1 day.

MAKES 5 CUPS; 5 SERVINGS OR 10 PORTIONS

1 Each 1-Decadent-Disk portion (about $1/2$ cup) has: 100 calories, 3 g protein, 18 g carbohydrates, 2 g fat, trace saturated fat, trace cholesterol, 2 g fiber, 210 mg sodium

2 Each 2-Decadent-Disk serving (about 1 cup) has: 201 calories, 5 g protein, 37 g carbohydrates, 4 g fat, <1 g saturated fat, <1 mg cholesterol, 3 g fiber, 421 mg sodium

You save: 238 calories, 29 g fat, 5 g saturated fat

Traditional serving: 439 calories, 9 g protein, 27 g carbohydrates, 33 g fat, 6 g saturated fat, 287 mg cholesterol, 4 g fiber, 833 mg sodium

entrées

IF YOU'RE LIKE MANY BUSY FOLKS, you're likely to have fallen into a food rut in the kitchen at some point over the years; you cook (or cooked) the same meals over and over. Then when you crave something out-of-the-box, so to speak, you rely on takeout, which isn't necessarily all that good for you.

Here's a full chapter (you'll notice that it's significantly larger than any other) that will satisfy your cravings from the privacy of your own home for a fraction of the fat and calories of most outside options. You can have Chinese tonight, followed by Italian tomorrow, then Mexican, Mediterranean, Cajun, English, even good old all-American mac and cheese, and more. I've covered Super Bowl festivities, Fourth of July parties, chili night, Italian Sunday dinner, and even Thanksgiving dinner. You can treat your family or even impress your boss with these simple, scrumptious meals, many of which can be prepared in minutes. You'll definitely save money and if you repurpose the decadent leftovers, you'll even end up saving time too.

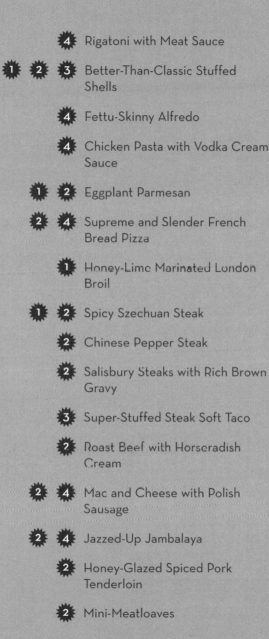

- **4** Rigatoni with Meat Sauce
- **1 2 3** Better-Than-Classic Stuffed Shells
- **4** Fettu-Skinny Alfredo
- **4** Chicken Pasta with Vodka Cream Sauce
- **1 2** Eggplant Parmesan
- **2 4** Supreme and Slender French Bread Pizza
- **1** Honey-Lime Marinated London Broil
- **1 2** Spicy Szechuan Steak
- **2** Chinese Pepper Steak
- **2** Salisbury Steaks with Rich Brown Gravy
- **3** Super-Stuffed Steak Soft Taco
- **2** Roast Beef with Horseradish Cream
- **2 4** Mac and Cheese with Polish Sausage
- **2 4** Jazzed-Up Jambalaya
- **2** Honey-Glazed Spiced Pork Tenderloin
- **2** Mini-Meatloaves

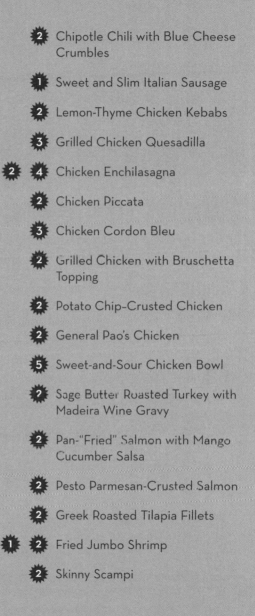

- **2** Chipotle Chili with Blue Cheese Crumbles
- **1** Sweet and Slim Italian Sausage
- **2** Lemon-Thyme Chicken Kebabs
- **3** Grilled Chicken Quesadilla
- **2 4** Chicken Enchilasagna
- **2** Chicken Piccata
- **3** Chicken Cordon Bleu
- **2** Grilled Chicken with Bruschetta Topping
- **2** Potato Chip–Crusted Chicken
- **2** General Pao's Chicken
- **5** Sweet-and-Sour Chicken Bowl
- **2** Sage Butter Roasted Turkey with Madeira Wine Gravy
- **2** Pan-"Fried" Salmon with Mango Cucumber Salsa
- **2** Pesto Parmesan-Crusted Salmon
- **2** Greek Roasted Tilapia Fillets
- **1 2** Fried Jumbo Shrimp
- **2** Skinny Scampi

RIGATONI WITH MEAT SAUCE

Rigatoni always makes me think of my grandmother on my dad's side. Gram is not the grandmother who taught me to cook—she was much more secretive with her recipes. But nearly every time we went to her house as kids, she had a huge pot of rigatoni and meatballs waiting for my dad. This is not actually Gram's recipe, but it's one that's requested often by my friends, especially now that carbs are no longer considered "bad." By adding plenty of lean meat sauce to the pasta, I end up with a perfectly balanced and scrumptious favorite.

If you're a fan of whole-wheat pasta, brown rice pasta, or any other variety containing fiber, I strongly encourage you to substitute that for the traditional penne. If you are newer to healthier eating and haven't converted to a fiber-rich pasta, that's okay too. It's all about making small changes that you can live with for the long haul.

8 ounces dried rigatoni pasta
$^3/_4$ pound 96% lean ground beef
1 teaspoon fennel seeds
$^1/_2$ teaspoon salt
$^1/_4$ teaspoon crushed red pepper flakes
$^1/_4$ teaspoon garlic powder
3 cups Mostly Mom's Marinara Sauce (recipe follows)
2 tablespoons grated reduced-fat Parmesan, divided

Cook the pasta according to package directions.

Mix the beef, fennel seeds, salt, red pepper flakes, and garlic powder in a medium bowl until well combined.

Place a large nonstick skillet over medium-high heat. When the skillet is hot, put in the beef mixture. Use a wooden spoon to break it into hearty chunks and cook until no longer pink inside, 2 to 4 minutes. Stir in the marinara sauce until warm.

Divide the pasta among 4 pasta bowls (about 1$^1/_2$ cups each). Top each with a quarter of the meat sauce (about a scant cup each). Sprinkle 1$^1/_2$ teaspoons Parmesan over the top of each. Serve immediately.

Can be made in 30 minutes or less

MAKES ABOUT 6 CUPS; 4 SERVINGS

 Each 4-Decadent-Disk serving ($^1/_4$ recipe) has: 404 calories, 29 g protein, 62 g carbohydrates, 6 g fat, 2 g saturated fat, 49 mg cholesterol, 6 g fiber, 777 mg sodium

You save: 181 calories, 17 g fat, 9 g saturated fat

Traditional serving: 585 calories, 29 g protein, 65 g carbohydrates, 23 g fat, 11 g saturated fat, 70 mg cholesterol, 5 g fiber, 1,136 mg sodium

MOSTLY MOM'S MARINARA SAUCE

Most people have their family-favorite marinara sauce—the one they grew up with. In my house, I had my grandmother Nan's sauce that we ate at holidays and when she visited. And then I had my mother's, which I also very much looked forward to.

This version is very similar to my mom's and evokes happy childhood memories for me. If your family recipe happens to be very low in fat (many marinaras are not, contrary to popular belief), use that as a substitute for this one. But if it has a significant amount of olive oil or other fat, you'll want to use this one or a low-fat, relatively low-sodium version.

Do note, however, that canned tomatoes contain different amounts of sugar and salt, depending on which brand you buy and even the time of year the tomatoes are packed. Thus you may need to alter the added salt and sugar each time you make this recipe to make it suit your taste. Just be sure to add as little as possible—you don't want to overdo it.

1 teaspoon extra virgin olive oil
1¹/₂ cups finely chopped onions
2 tablespoons minced fresh garlic
Two 28-ounce cans crushed tomatoes
1 tablespoon dried oregano
2 teaspoons sugar, plus extra, if desired
¹/₂ teaspoon crushed red pepper flakes
¹/₂ teaspoon salt, or to taste

Place a large nonstick saucepan over medium heat. Put in the olive oil, onions, and garlic. Cook, stirring occasionally, until tender but not brown, 7 to 10 minutes. Add the crushed tomatoes, oregano, sugar, red pepper flakes, and ¹/₂ teaspoon salt. Stir until well combined. Turn the heat to low. Cook, covered, for at least 1 hour, stirring occasionally. Season with additional salt, if needed.

MAKES 6¹/₂ TO 7 CUPS
Each ¹/₂-cup serving has: 55 calories, 2 g protein, 12 g carbohydrates, <1 g fat, trace saturated fat, 0 mg cholesterol, 3 g fiber, 252 mg sodium

BETTER-THAN-CLASSIC STUFFED SHELLS

1 **2** **3**

Over the years, I've heard so many people say that fat-free ricotta cheese doesn't taste good. Although I agree that many dishes made with it do not, this is definitely not one of them. In fact, this is one of the dishes I serve to friends who claim they would never eat lower-fat food, because it fools them every time. When the fat-free ricotta is combined with the other ingredients, you'd never ever guess that this was made with lower-fat anything. It's the perfect dish for entertaining—and I know. I've served it time and time again.

You may notice as you flip through this book that I rarely use fat-free products. I almost always choose low-fat or light. So trust me, if I thought the fat-free didn't taste out of this world in this recipe (I use Precious or Sorrento brands), I would have picked light here, too.

12 dried jumbo pasta shells

1 cup fat-free ricotta cheese

4 ounces (about 1¼ cups) finely shredded low-fat mozzarella (2½ grams of fat or less per ounce)

3 tablespoons grated reduced-fat Parmesan, divided

1 large egg white

1½ teaspoons finely chopped fresh parsley

¼ teaspoon garlic powder

Salt and pepper

2 cups Mostly Mom's Marinara Sauce (page 101) or other low-fat, low-sodium marinara sauce

Preheat the oven to 350°F.

Cook the pasta according to package directions, cooking it only al dente. Drain and reserve.

Place a sheet of wax paper large enough to hold 12 filled shells on a flat work surface.

Mix the ricotta, mozzarella, 2 tablespoons Parmesan, egg white, parsley, and garlic powder in a medium bowl. Season with salt and pepper to taste.

Place the cooked shells, open side up, on the wax paper. Spoon the ricotta mixture evenly among them, about 2 heaping tablespoons in each.

Evenly spread about ½ cup marinara sauce in a 10-inch round or an 11 X 7-inch ovenproof glass baking dish, or a casserole dish large enough to hold the stuffed shells in a single layer. Lay the stuffed shells side by side, open side up, in the dish. Spoon the remaining marinara sauce over the top. Then sprinkle the remaining Parmesan evenly over the marinara sauce. Cover with foil and bake for 20 to 25 minutes. Let stand for 5 minutes before serving.

MAKES 12 SHELLS; 4 SERVINGS OR 6 OR 12 PORTIONS

1 Each 1-Decadent-Disk portion (1 shell) has: 99 calories, 7 g protein, 14 g carbohydrates, 2 g fat, trace saturated fat, 9 mg cholesterol, 2 g fiber, 205 mg sodium

2 Each 2-Decadent-Disk portion (2 shells) has: 197 calories, 13 g protein, 29 g carbohydrates, 3 g fat, <1 g saturated fat, 17 mg cholesterol, 3 g fiber, 410 mg sodium

3 Each 3-Decadent-Disk serving (3 shells) has: 296 calories, 20 g protein, 43 g carbohydrates, 5 g fat, 1 g saturated fat, 26 mg cholesterol, 5 g fiber, 615 mg sodium

Better-Than-Classic Stuffed Shells
with Fried Zucchini (page 183)

FETTU-SKINNY ALFREDO

When I was growing up, we always vacationed in Stone Harbor, New Jersey. There was an amazing little Italian restaurant where we would go often. It's probably the only Italian restaurant I've ever been to where I thought the food was arguably as good as my Italian grandmother's. I loved their meatballs and loved, loved, loved their fettuccine Alfredo. In fact, I loved them so much, I couldn't wait to go back "to the shore" every summer for that alone. Now I have this grown-up, guilt-free twist that is so much leaner it's insane.

This dish, made as directed, has more than enough sauce to coat the pasta, so if you're like me and like to have plenty of protein at each meal, adding shrimp or extra-lean grilled chicken is a great option, For another 100 calories, you can add 3^1/$_2$ ounces of grilled shrimp or extra-lean grilled chicken. And if you want to make the dish even leaner, omit a little bit of the butter. It's still rich and creamy without it; it just won't have that really buttery taste.

9 ounces dried fettuccine
2^1/$_2$ teaspoons unbleached all-purpose flour
1 cup plus 2 tablespoons fat-free half-and-half
^{1}/$_2$ cup plus 2 tablespoons grated reduced-fat
    Parmesan, divided

^{1}/$_2$ teaspoon garlic powder, or more to taste
^{1}/$_8$ teaspoon salt, or to taste
3 tablespoons light butter (stick, not tub)
Chopped fresh parsley, optional

Cook the fettuccine according to package directions.

Mix the flour with just enough half-and-half to form a paste in a medium bowl. Slowly add the remaining half-and-half, stirring to remove any lumps.

Place a medium nonstick skillet over medium heat. Put in the half-and-half mixture, ^{1}/$_2$ cup Parmesan, the garlic powder, and salt to taste. Cook, stirring constantly, until the mixture is as thick as a gravy, 5 to 7 minutes. Stir in the butter until it melts and is well incorporated. Toss in the cooked fettuccine. If the sauce still needs to thicken slightly, continue to toss the fettuccine until the sauce thickens. Divide the fettuccine among 4 pasta bowls or dinner plates. Top each with 1^1/$_2$ teaspoons of the remaining Parmesan and a sprinkling of parsley, if desired. Serve immediately.

Can be made in 30 minutes or less / No more than 20 minutes hands-on prep time

MAKES 5 CUPS; 4 SERVINGS

Each 4-Decadent-Disk serving (1^1/$_4$ cups) has: 397 calories, 13 g protein, 64 g carbohydrates, 9 g fat, 3 g saturated fat, 11 mg cholesterol, 2 g fiber, 485 mg sodium

You save: 222 calories, 22 g fat, 16 g saturated fat

Traditional serving: 619 calories, 22 g protein, 63 g carbohydrates, 31 g fat, 19 g saturated fat, 95 mg cholesterol, 0 g fiber, 1,080 mg sodium

CHICKEN PASTA WITH VODKA CREAM SAUCE

4

I created this recipe at the request of one of my celebrity clients. She was trying to lose weight for a movie and swore she kept having nightmares about having overeaten pasta with vodka sauce. She thought I wouldn't be able to redesign it because it's a cream-based sauce. But I managed to quell her craving—and her nightmares. I also suggested she add some chicken to the dish. Though I don't believe any foods are "bad," it's always great to add bulk to your meals with lean protein, especially when you're trying to build muscle. Who knew vodka and looking buff could go hand in hand?

1¹/2 cups Vodka Cream Sauce (recipe follows)

8 ounces dried enriched multigrain rotini or penne pasta

12 ounces boneless, skinless chicken breast, visible fat removed, cut into ³/4-inch-wide strips

1¹/2 teaspoons extra virgin olive oil

Salt and pepper

2 teaspoons grated reduced-fat Parmesan

4 tablespoons slivered fresh basil leaves, or to taste (see page 20)

Prepare the Vodka Cream Sauce.

Cook the pasta according to package directions.

Toss the chicken and olive oil in a small bowl, and season with salt and pepper to taste.

Place a medium nonstick skillet over medium-high heat. When the skillet is hot, put in the chicken and cook until browned on the outside and no longer pink inside, about 3 minutes per side.

Drain the pasta and divide it among 4 medium shallow bowls. Spoon a quarter of the sauce into the center of each. Top each bowl with a quarter of the chicken. Then sprinkle a quarter of the Parmesan and basil leaves evenly over the top of each bowl. Serve immediately. *(continued)*

MAKES 4 SERVINGS

4 Each 4-Decadent-Disk serving (¹/4 recipe) has: 401 calories, 33 g protein, 50 g carbohydrates, 6 g fat, <1 g saturated fat, 55 mg cholesterol, 6 g fiber, 349 mg sodium

VODKA CREAM SAUCE

Vodka cream sauce does have vodka in it, but not a lot. It's actually a creamy tomato sauce with the mildest hint of vodka. When you make this, I implore you to chop the garlic yourself—the stuff in the jar just won't give you the same flavor. If you're short on time, just buy the peeled cloves that are now found in the produce section of most major grocery stores. They can be chopped in seconds.

1 teaspoon extra virgin olive oil
1 cup minced sweet onions
1 tablespoon minced or crushed fresh garlic
One 28-ounce can crushed tomatoes
$^{1}/_{3}$ cup vodka
1 cup fat-free half-and-half
2 teaspoons fresh lemon juice
$^{1}/_{4}$ cup plus 2 tablespoons reduced-fat Parmesan
$^{1}/_{2}$ teaspoon dried basil
$^{1}/_{2}$ teaspoon dried oregano
1 teaspoon sugar
$^{1}/_{4}$ teaspoon salt

Place a medium nonstick saucepan over medium heat. Put in the olive oil, onions, and garlic and cook, stirring occasionally, until the onions and garlic are sweating and tender but not at all browned, 8 to 10 minutes.

Reduce the heat to low. Add the tomatoes and vodka. Slowly stir in the half-and-half. Then stir in the lemon juice, Parmesan, basil, oregano, sugar, and salt until smooth and well combined. Cook over the lowest heat setting, covered, for at least 3 hours, stirring occasionally. Serve immediately, or refrigerate in an airtight container for up to 5 days.

Makes approximately 4 cups; 8 servings
Each $^{1}/_{2}$-cup serving has: 111 calories, 4 g protein, 15 g carbohydrates, 2 g fat, trace saturated fat, 7 mg cholesterol, 2 g fiber, 332 mg sodium

EGGPLANT PARMESAN

1   **2**

My lead assistant, Stephanie, is a vegetarian. I don't know how she does it (I'm such a meat-and-potatoes lover myself). She enjoys cooking for her boyfriend, Andy, and this is one of their faves.

When I recently served this dish at a dinner party, I was surprised how many of the guests were excited about it, particularly because most chefs highly salt the eggplant to remove moisture before breading it. Here, we saved some sodium and still managed great results.

Please note that it is very important that during the initial baking of the eggplant, you don't layer the slices on top of one another. If you do, they will not brown. Oh, and be sure to have the cheese already shredded before you begin layering the eggplant, sauce, and cheese to prevent the eggplant from getting soggy. You, too, will be more than satisfied with this tasty, seemingly fattening dish.

Olive oil spray

2 large egg whites

1 teaspoon fat-free milk

$^{2}/_{3}$ cup dried bread crumbs

$^{1}/_{4}$ teaspoon garlic powder

1 teaspoon finely chopped fresh parsley

$^{1}/_{8}$ teaspoon salt

1 pound eggplant, cut crosswise into $^{1}/_{4}$-inch circles

1$^{1}/_{2}$ cups Mostly Mom's Marinara Sauce (page 101) or other low-fat, low-sodium marinara sauce, divided

4 ounces (about 1$^{1}/_{4}$ cups) finely shredded low-fat mozzarella (2$^{1}/_{2}$ grams of fat or less per ounce)

1 tablespoon grated reduced-fat Parmesan

Preheat the oven to 400°F.

Mist a large nonstick baking sheet (or sheets) with spray.

Use a fork to lightly beat the egg whites and milk in a medium shallow bowl until well combined.

Combine the bread crumbs, garlic powder, parsley, and salt in a second medium shallow bowl and set it next to the first.   *(continued)*

MAKES 1 CASSEROLE; 4 SERVINGS OR 8 PORTIONS

1 Each 1-Decadent-Disk portion ($^{1}/_{8}$ casserole) has: 102 calories, 7 g protein, 13 g carbohydrates, 2 g fat, <1 g saturated fat, 6 mg cholesterol, 3 g fiber, 273 mg sodium

2 Each 2-Decadent-Disk serving ($^{1}/_{4}$ casserole) has: 204 calories, 14 g protein, 26 g carbohydrates, 5 g fat, 1 g saturated fat, 12 mg cholesterol, 6 g fiber, 547 mg sodium

You save: 250 calories, 27 g fat, 13 g saturated fat

Traditional serving: 454 calories, 19 g protein, 26 g carbohydrates, 32 g fat, 14 g saturated fat, 66 mg cholesterol, 5 g fiber, 593 mg sodium

Dip one of the eggplant slices into the egg mixture, letting any excess drip off. Next, dip the eggplant into the bread crumb mixture and lay it on a prepared baking sheet. Continue breading the remaining eggplant slices, laying them side by side, not touching, on the baking sheets. Transfer the sheets to the oven rack (bake one after the other if they do not fit side by side on one rack) and bake for 10 to 12 minutes. Carefully flip the slices and bake for another 10 to 12 minutes, until the eggplant is lightly browned and the breading is crisp. Remove from the oven and reduce the oven temperature to 350°F.

Meanwhile, spread $1/2$ cup marinara sauce evenly over the bottom of an 11 X 7-inch baking dish. Layer half of the eggplant slices on top of the marinara sauce (it's okay if they overlap a little). Spoon another $1/2$ cup of the marinara sauce evenly over the eggplant, followed by half of the mozzarella. Layer the remaining eggplant slices over the mozzarella, followed by another $1/2$ cup of marinara sauce and the remaining mozzarella. Sprinkle the tops evenly with the Parmesan. Bake, uncovered, for 20 to 25 minutes, or until the cheese is bubbly and beginning to brown slightly. Serve immediately.

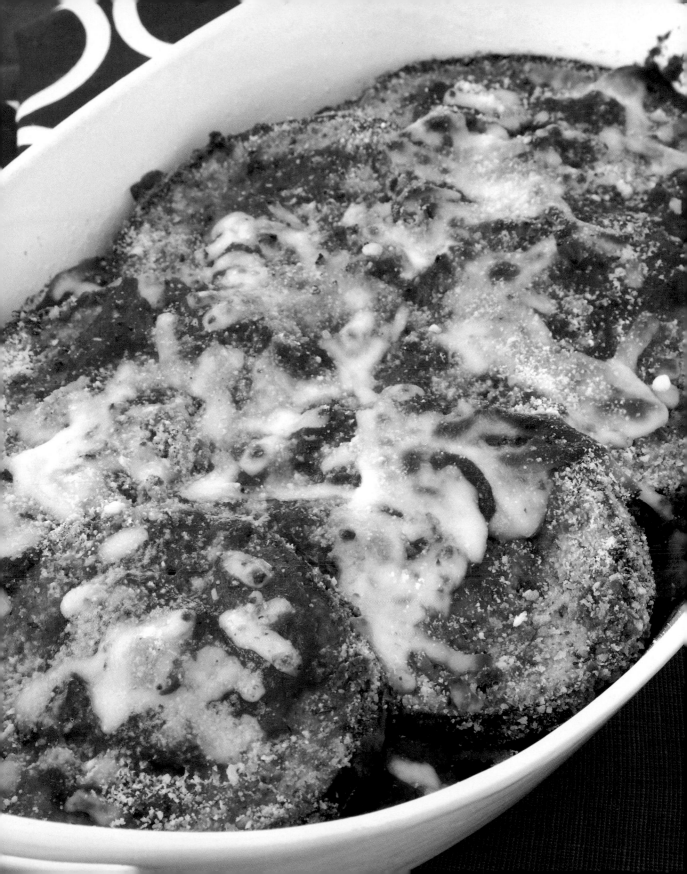

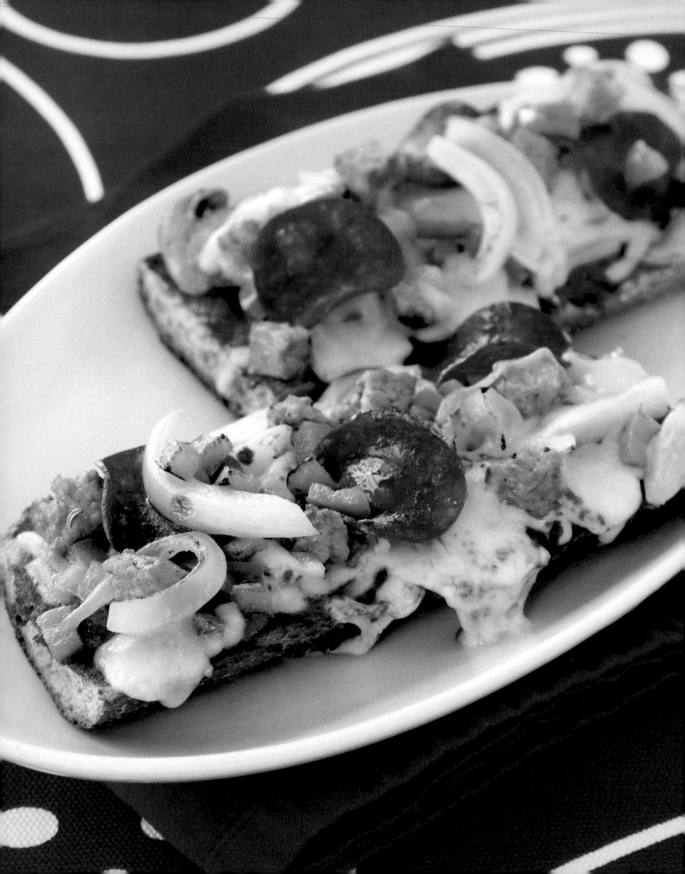

SUPREME AND SLENDER FRENCH BREAD PIZZA

2 **4**

Almost everyone I know grew up eating the French bread pizza you find in freezers at the grocery store. Even people who don't otherwise eat frozen foods tend to have happy memories associated with it. I not only indulged in it often, I made it myself, even as a kid. The problem is that it's so greasy most of the time, especially if you add the best toppings like pepperoni and sausage. Here I've tweaked it, adding some fiber by using a whole grain baguette, and using much lighter versions of pepperoni, sausage, and cheese. And I always shred the cheese finely. Not only does it mean that you need less to cover the entire surface of the pizza, it will melt better, more closely mimicking full-fat cheese.

Please note that any time you're making pizza, it's important to paritally cook any veggies like mushrooms, onions or bell peppers, which have a high moisture content. If you don't, the liquid released from them will make the pizza crust soggy. Also, this recipe is high in sodium and there is no way to eliminate it without eliminating major amounts of flavor. Just be wary of that so you don't over do it over the course of the day.

One 3-ounce-piece (5 to 6 inches) multi-grain or
   whole wheat French baguette
Olive oil spray
$^1/_3$ cup onion slivers
3 tablespoons chopped green bell pepper
2 medium button mushrooms, sliced

$^1/_4$ cup Mostly Mom's Marinara Sauce (page 101) or
   other low-fat, low-sodium pizza or marinara
   sauce
1 ounce (about $^1/_4$ cup plus 1 tablespoon) finely
   shredded low-fat mozzarella cheese
Fresh or dried oregano leaves, to taste (optional)
Crushed red pepper flakes (optional)
1 ounce ($^1/_2$ link) Sweet and Slim Italian Sausage
   (page 130), coarsely chopped
6 slices turkey pepperoni

Preheat the oven to 400° F.

Cut the baguette in half lengthwise. Place the halves on a nonstick baking sheet, insides faceup. Bake them for 5 to 7 minutes, until lightly toasted.

Meanwhile, lightly mist a small skillet with spray and place it over medium heat. Add the onions, peppers, and mushrooms and cook them about 5 minutes, stirring occasionally, until just tender, but not brown.

Top the toasted baguette evenly with the marinara sauce, then half of the onion mxture, then the cheese. Sprinkle evenly with oregano and crushed red pepper flakes, if using. Place the sausage and pepperoni over that, followed by the remaining onion mixture. Return the pizza to the oven and bake until the cheese is just melted and the bread is crisp, about 5 to 8 minutes. Serve immediately.

MAKES 2 PIECES; 1 SERVING OR 2 PORTIONS

2 Each 2-Decadent-Disk portion (1 piece) has: 197 calories, 12 g protein, 29 g carbohydrates,
4 g fat, <1 saturated fat, 19 mg cholesterol, 3 g fiber, 549 mg sodium

4 Each 4-Decadent-Disk serving (2 pieces) has: 396 calories, 26 g protein, 56 g carbohydrates,
8 g fat, 2 g saturated fat, 37 mg cholesterol, 7 g fiber, 991 mg sodium

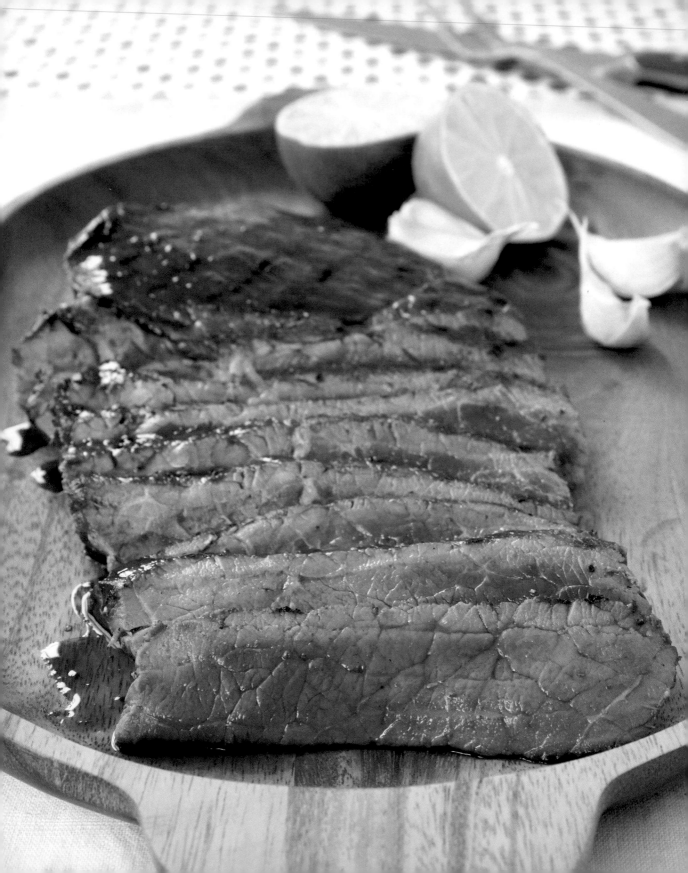

HONEY-LIME MARINATED LONDON BROIL

⭐

We all know that Mexican food tends to be on the very heavy side. I try to avoid eating at Mexican restaurants even though they house some of my all-time favorite flavors. This recipe is much more subtle in flavor than most in this book and much leaner than many other marinades with a Mexican flair. It makes the leftovers a great option for so many other dishes—salads, sandwiches, quesadillas, and tacos—with a fraction of the sodium, fat, and calories normally found in these dishes.

¹/₄ cup fresh lime juice

2 tablespoons extra virgin olive oil

1 tablespoon plus 1 teaspoon honey

2 tablespoons minced fresh garlic

1 teaspoon salt

1¹/₄ pounds trimmed London broil (top round steak)

Whisk the lime juice, olive oil, and honey in a small bowl. Stir in the garlic and salt.

Place the steak in a large resealable plastic bag. Pour in the marinade. Seal the bag and rotate it so the steak is covered with the marinade. Place the bag in the refrigerator and marinate the steak for at least 6 hours or overnight, rotating it occasionally, if possible.

Preheat a grill to high.

Remove the steak from the marinade and place it on the grill. Discard the remaining marinade. Grill for 4 to 6 minutes per side for medium-rare, or until the desired doneness is reached. Place the steak on a plate or cutting board, cover loosely with foil, and let stand for 10 minutes. Slice into thin slices against the grain and serve immediately, or refrigerate the uncut steak in an airtight container and slice it just before serving.

No more than 20 minutes hands-on prep time

MAKES 6 PORTIONS

⭐ Each 1-Decadent-Disk portion (about 3 ounces) has: 107 calories, 20 g protein, 1 g carbohydrates, 4 g fat, 1 g saturated fat, 42 mg cholesterol, <1 g fiber, 143 mg sodium

SPICY SZECHUAN STEAK

1 **2**

Even though I'm a chef and arguably quicker than many at throwing dinner together, sometimes I just don't feel like spending extra time in the kitchen. This steak is a great solution. It takes seconds to make the marinade, so I can come home to a ready-to-grill entrée that can be on the table in less than 15 minutes.

When I'm finished eating, I pack the leftovers. The next day, I slice the steak and eat it cold as deli meat or use it to top salads. It's just as great that way and I don't have to cook again. Plus, I save tons of calories, fat, sodium, and even money over eating out.

2 tablespoons bottled Szechuan sauce
2 teaspoons minced fresh garlic
1¹/₂ teaspoons olive oil
1 teaspoon black pepper
1¹/₂ pounds trimmed London broil (top round steak)

Stir together the Szechuan sauce, garlic, olive oil, and pepper in a small bowl. Rub the mixture evenly over the steak and transfer it to a large resealable plastic bag. Seal the bag and refrigerate for at least 4 hours or overnight.

Preheat a grill to high.

Remove the steak from the bag and place it on the grill. Grill for 5 minutes per side for medium-rare, or until the desired doneness is reached. Place the steak on a platter, cover loosely with foil, and let stand for 10 minutes. Slice into thin slices against the grain and serve immediately, or refrigerate the uncut steak and slice it just before serving.

No more than 20 minutes hands-on prep time

MAKES 4 SERVINGS OR 8 PORTIONS

1 Each 1-Decadent-Disk portion (2¹/₂ ounces) has: 97 calories, 18 g protein, 1 g carbohydrates, 4 g fat, 1 g saturated fat, 38 mg cholesterol, trace fiber, 96 mg sodium

2 Each 2-Decadent-Disk serving (5 ounces) has: 195 calories, 36 g protein, 2 g carbohydrates, 7 g fat, 3 g saturated fat, 75 mg cholesterol, trace fiber, 192 mg sodium

CHINESE PEPPER STEAK

In addition to loving this dish served hot from the stove, it's become one of my favorites because it makes such excellent leftovers. Toss it on some rice for a complete meal then save some to reheat in the microwave at work the next day, and your co-workers are sure to be jealous.

Please note: the meat is cooked in batches so it browns properly and ends up being tender.

1¹/₂ pounds trimmed top round steak, cut into ¹/₂-inch-thick strips

1 teaspoon black pepper

¹/₂ teaspoon garlic powder

¹/₄ teaspoon salt

3¹/₂ teaspoons extra virgin olive oil, divided

1¹/₂ cups ¹/₂-inch-wide, 2-inch-long sweet onion strips

1¹/₄ cups ¹/₂-inch-wide, 2-inch-long green bell pepper strips (about 1 large pepper; see page 20)

1 teaspoon minced fresh garlic

2 cups canned crushed tomatoes

1¹/₂ tablespoons low-sodium soy sauce

Place the steak in a medium bowl. Add the black pepper, garlic powder, and salt. Toss to season the steak evenly. Let stand for 10 minutes.

Place a large nonstick saucepan over high heat. When the pan is hot, put in 1 teaspoon olive oil. Add half of the steak and brown it on all sides, 1 to 2 minutes per side. Remove from the pan. Add another teaspoon of olive oil, then the remaining steak. Brown that on all sides. Remove from the pan. Turn the heat to medium, and then add the remaining 1¹/₂ teaspoons olive oil, onion, bell pepper, and garlic. Cook, stirring occasionally, until just tender, about 5 minutes. Return the steak to the pan, and then stir in the tomatoes and soy sauce. Turn the heat back to high. When the liquid reaches a boil, cover the pan and turn the heat to low. Simmer, stirring occasionally, until the meat is tender enough to fall apart with a fork, about 1¹/₂ hours. Serve immediately, or refrigerate in an airtight container for up to 3 days.

MAKES ABOUT 6 CUPS; 6 SERVINGS

 Each 2-Decadent-Disk serving (1 cup) has: 192 calories, 26 g protein, 12 g carbohydrates, 6 g fat, 2 g saturated fat, 50 mg cholesterol, 3 g fiber, 480 mg sodium

SALISBURY STEAKS WITH RICH BROWN GRAVY

2

I have to admit I was pretty intimidated at the notion of making over Salisbury steak. But I've gotten numerous fan letters over the years with requests for it, so I knew I had to include it in this book.

I was worried that it would be tough to make a great, creamy gravy that wasn't full of fat or way too much salt. Many recipes for Salisbury steak call for an entire envelope of onion soup mix, which tends to have about 2,800 milligrams of sodium in just that ingredient. Others that don't include it have a laundry list of ingredients that would take way too long to prepare.

Ready for the challenge, I was pleasantly surprised with the results. I originally tried it with a bit more onion soup mix, but realized it could do without the added salt. I removed some and added dried minced onion. This way, you save sodium, but still get that deep onion flavor.

Because there is plenty of gravy, this dish is great served with egg noodles or Horseradish Smashed Potatoes (page 167). For another 100 calories, you can have $1/2$ cup of egg noodles or $1/3$ cup of Horseradish Smashed Potatoes.

$1/3$ cup egg substitute

$1/4$ cup old-fashioned oats

1 tablespoon plus 2 teaspoons onion soup mix

1 tablespoon dried minced onion

$1/2$ teaspoon garlic powder

$1/4$ teaspoon black pepper

1 pound 96% lean ground beef

3 tablespoons unbleached all-purpose flour, divided

1 cup fat-free, lower-sodium beef broth

2 tablespoons ketchup

2 teaspoons Worcestershire sauce

Olive oil spray

1 onion, sliced and separated into rings (about $3^{1}/2$ cups)

Can be made in 30 minutes or less / No more than 20 minutes hands-on prep time

MAKES 4 PATTIES; 4 SERVINGS

2 Each 2-Decadent-Disk serving (1 patty with $1/4$ of the gravy and onions) has: 205 calories, 26 g protein, 13 g carbohydrates, 5 g fat, 2 g saturated fat, 60 mg cholesterol, 1 g fiber, 573 mg sodium

You save: 126 calories, 14 g fat, 5 g saturated fat

Traditional serving: 331 calories, 25 g protein, 14 g carbohydrates, 19 g fat, 7 g saturated fat, 112 mg cholesterol, 1 g fiber, 818 mg sodium

Combine the egg substitute and the oats in a medium mixing bowl. Let stand for 3 minutes to soften the oats. Add the onion soup mix, minced onion, garlic powder, pepper, and beef. Mix until well combined, and then shape into 4 oval patties about 1 inch thick, 3 inches wide, and 4$\frac{1}{2}$ inches long.

Put 2 tablespoons of the flour in a medium shallow bowl. Dip the patties in the flour to coat them on all sides. Shake off any excess.

Put the remaining flour in a medium mixing bowl. Slowly whisk in enough broth to form a paste. Then slowly whisk in the remaining broth, then the ketchup and Worcestershire sauce until well combined. Set aside.

Preheat a large nonstick skillet to medium-high heat. When the skillet is hot, lightly mist it with spray. Put in the patties, side by side. Brown on both sides, 1 to 2 minutes per side. Pour the broth mixture into the skillet. Add the onion rings to the skillet. Use a wooden spoon to stir them gently into the broth mixture, being careful not to break the patties. Bring the liquid to a boil. Cover the pan, reduce the heat to low, and simmer for 15 minutes, flipping the patties once, halfway through. Transfer the patties to a platter. Spoon the onions and gravy over the patties. Serve immediately.

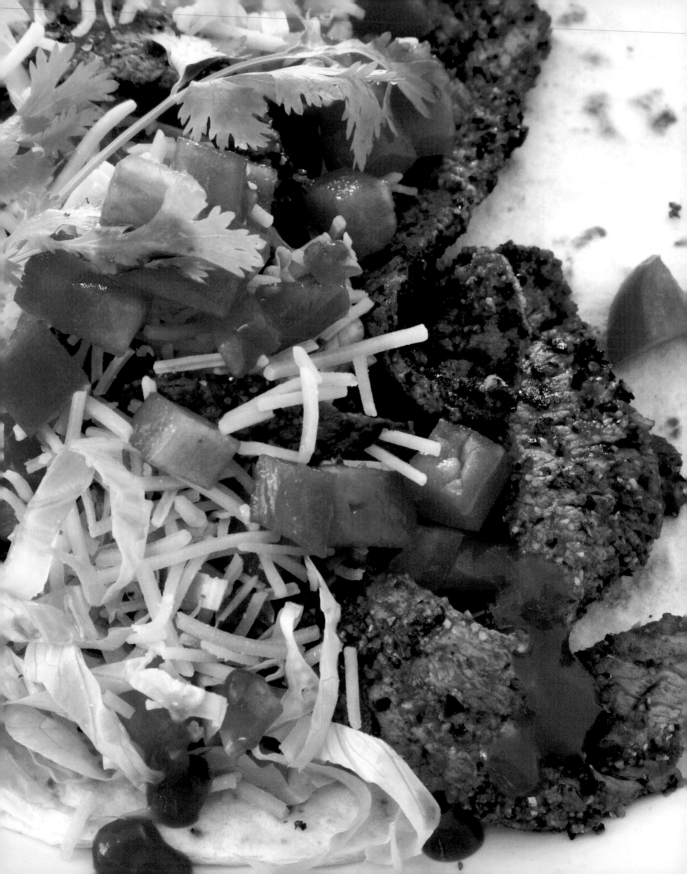

SUPER-STUFFED STEAK SOFT TACO

3

People often say that lean meat is tough. It's just not true if you cook it and cut it correctly. First, always start cooking it with high heat. When making a roast, you can sear the outsides, then cook it on low heat in the oven.

For a recipe like this where you're cooking strips of steak, start by tenderizing the meat with the toothed side of a meat mallet. Then make sure your pan is nice and hot, and don't overcrowd it with too much meat at once. It should get browned on the outside before overcooking on the inside. Next, when you cut meat, always cut it against the grain (see page 20).

Taco sauce has only about 5 calories per tablespoon, so as long as you don't go crazy with it, you can't go wrong using it to add even more flavor.

4 ounces top round steak
1 (about 8-inch diameter) low-carb flour tortilla
$^1/_2$ to 1 teaspoon salt-free Mexican or Southwest
   seasoning (see page 17)
$^1/_8$ teaspoon garlic powder
Pinch of salt, or to taste
Olive oil spray
$^2/_3$ cup finely shredded romaine lettuce
$^1/_4$ cup chopped tomato

1 ounce (about $^1/_2$ cup) finely shredded Cabot's
   75% Light Cheddar cheese, or your favorite
   low-fat Cheddar
Mild, medium, or hot red taco sauce
2 tablespoons fresh cilantro

Preheat the oven to 400°F.

Place the steak between two sheets of plastic wrap or wax paper on a flat work surface. Use the toothed side of a meat mallet to pound both sides of the steak to tenderize it, until it is about $^1/_3$ inch thick. Cut it into $^1/_4$-inch strips.

Wrap the tortilla in aluminum foil so that it is completely covered. Place the foil directly on the oven rack and heat the tortilla until warm, 5 to 7 minutes.

Mix the Mexican seasoning, garlic powder, and salt in a medium bowl. Add the steak strips and toss to coat evenly.

Preheat a small nonstick skillet to medium-high heat. When the skillet is hot, mist it lightly with spray. Add the steak strips in a single layer and cook, stirring occasionally, just until the outsides are browned and the insides are pink, 2 to 4 minutes.

Place the tortilla on a plate. Evenly spoon the steak strips over half. Top evenly with the lettuce, tomato, cheese, taco sauce, and cilantro. Fold the bare half over. Serve immediately.

Can be made in 30 minutes or less / No more than 20 minutes hands-on prep time

MAKES 1 TACO; 1 SERVING

3 Each 3-Decadent-Disk serving (1 taco) has: 299 calories, 39 g protein, 22 g carbohydrates, 9 g fat, 4 g saturated fat, 60 mg cholesterol, 12 g fiber, 666 mg sodium

Roast Beef with Horseradish Cream and
Parmesan-Garlic Mashed Potato Pancakes (page 164)

ROAST BEEF WITH HORSERADISH CREAM

2

Bar none, one of the best parts of my job is showing meat-and-potatoes lovers that they can still eat their favorite foods and be healthy. I'm a meat-and-potatoes gal myself, so I can relate to not wanting to (or being able to) give them up. Here you don't have to. You can treat your family to the ultimate meat-and-potatoes feast. And the best part? The leftover roast beef can be sliced extremely thin and used for sandwiches that will save you tons of sodium over traditional deli meats. Note: the thinner you slice it, the more tender it will be in your sandwiches.

Be sure to drain the horseradish well. Simply put it in a fine sieve, and then use a spoon to press it gently until no more liquid is released. Doing this will ensure a thick, creamy sauce. Also, if at all possible, use sea salt for this recipe. Since it's so integral in flavoring the roast, you don't want to skimp and use plain old table salt.

$1/2$ teaspoon onion powder
$1/4$ teaspoon garlic powder
$1/2$ to 1 teaspoon sea salt
$1/2$ to 1 teaspoon freshly ground black pepper
$2^1/4$ pounds trimmed beef eye round roast (weight after all visible fat is removed)
$1^1/2$ teaspoons extra virgin olive oil
1 recipe Horseradish Cream (recipe follows)

Mix together the onion powder, garlic powder, and salt and pepper, to taste, in a small bowl until well combined.

Preheat the oven to 350°F.

Rub the entire roast evenly with the olive oil. Then rub the salt mixture into the roast to cover it entirely. Let stand for 20 minutes.

Meanwhile, make the Horseradish Cream.

Place a medium nonstick skillet over high heat. When the skillet is hot, put in the roast and cook for 1 to 2 minutes per side, including each end, until just browned all over. Then transfer the roast to a medium nonstick roasting pan and place in the center of the oven. Roast for 40 to 45 minutes, until a meat thermometer inserted in the center reaches about 125°F for medium-rare (the temperature will rise another 5° to 10°F while standing), or until the desired doneness is reached. Remove the roast from the oven and transfer it to a platter. Loosely cover the roast with foil and let stand for 10 to 15 minutes. Slice thinly and serve immediately with Horseradish Cream, or refrigerate for up to 3 days and slice thinly just before serving. *(continued)*

No more than 20 minutes hands-on prep time

MAKES 8 SERVINGS

2 Each 2-Decadent-Disk serving (4 ounces roast with 2 tablespoons Horseradish Cream) has: 202 calories, 29 g protein, 5 g carbohydrates, 7 g fat, 3 g saturated fat, 62 mg cholesterol, trace fiber, 233 mg sodium

HORSERADISH CREAM

3 tablespoons bottled horseradish, or more to
   taste
1 cup light sour cream
$1/4$ cup minced green onion tops
Salt and pepper

Spoon the horseradish into a fine strainer. Use the back of a spoon to gently press it to release excess moisture. Stir and continue pressing until liquid no longer drips from it. Transfer to a medium bowl. Add the sour cream and green onion, and then whisk until well combined. Season with salt and pepper to taste. Cover and refrigerate for 2 hours to 2 days.

Makes about 1 cup; 8 servings
Each 2-tablespoon serving has: 39 calories,
1 g protein, 5 g carbohydrates, 2 g fat, 2 g saturated
fat, 10 mg cholesterol, trace fiber, 49 mg sodium

MAC AND CHEESE WITH POLISH SAUSAGE

One day I was hanging out with my friend Jon, and he told me he always made mac and cheese with smoked sausage for his daughter, Justice. Apparently, it is one of her all-time favorite dishes. Being a single dad, he loved making it because he said it was super-easy. I, of course, was a little worried about the fat and sodium content in the version he was serving, so I developed this one. Justice loved this one, too!

Note that you can use any brand of turkey smoked sausage or kielbasa that you like. Just be sure to get the leanest one you can find. I use one that has 3 grams of fat per 2-ounce serving (see page 17), and it's absolutely delicious. You can also use any brand of Cheddar that you love that has $2^{1}/_{2}$ grams of fat or less per ounce. I use Cabot's because it's lighter than most, melts very well, and has a genuine Cheddar taste.

4 ounces extra-lean kielbasa or smoked turkey
    sausage (3 grams of fat or less per 2-ounce
    serving)
1 cup dried elbow macaroni
2 teaspoons unbleached all-purpose flour

$^{1}/_{4}$ cup fat-free milk
$^{1}/_{8}$ teaspoon salt
$3^{1}/_{2}$ ounces ($1^{3}/_{4}$ cups) finely shredded Cabot's
    75% Light Cheddar cheese, or your favorite
    low-fat Cheddar

Bring a medium pot of lightly salted water to a full boil.

Cut the sausage into $^{1}/_{4}$-inch-thick slices.

Add the macaroni and the sausage to the pot and cook, stirring occasionally, until the macaroni is cooked al dente, about 5 minutes. (It should still have a bit of bite to it.) Drain.

Meanwhile, mix the flour with just enough milk to form a paste in a small bowl. Slowly add the remaining milk, stirring as you do, making sure to remove any lumps. Place a medium saucepan over medium heat. Pour the milk mixture into the saucepan. Stir in the salt. Add the cheese and continue to stir the mixture with a wooden spoon until the cheese is completely melted and the mixture starts to thicken. When the mixture is almost smooth, stir in the cooked macaroni and sausage until it is well incorporated. Serve immediately.

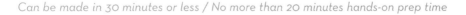

Can be made in 30 minutes or less / No more than 20 minutes hands-on prep time

MAKES 3 CUPS; 2 SERVINGS OR 4 PORTIONS

Each 2-Decadent-Disk portion ($^{3}/_{4}$ cup) has: 199 calories, 17 g protein, 24 g carbohydrates, 4 g fat, 2 g saturated fat, 27 mg cholesterol, 1 g fiber, 550 mg sodium

Each 4-Decadent-Disk serving ($1^{1}/_{2}$ cups) has: 397 calories, 34 g protein, 47 g carbohydrates, 9 g fat, 4 g saturated fat, 53 mg cholesterol, 2 g fiber, 1,101 mg sodium

You save: 305 calories, 33 g fat, 20 g saturated fat

Traditional serving: 702 calories, 32 g protein, 48 g carbohydrates, 42 g fat, 24 g saturated fat, 120 mg cholesterol, 2 g fiber, 1,738 mg sodium

JAZZED-UP JAMBALAYA

2 **4**

Oh boy, do I love jambalaya. If I could eat it every day, I probably would. I love spicy food, shrimp, and sausage. This dish combines all of those flavors, and it's one that I often cook.

Though jambalaya most often uses smoked sausage or ham, I use turkey smoked sausage or turkey kielbasa. If you're not familiar with it, kielbasa is a Polish smoked sausage. In a dish like this, it tastes very similar to American smoked sausage. The varieties I use have only 3 grams of fat for 2 ounces and taste great (see page 17). You'd never guess they're as light as they are. Always check labels; a few brands of turkey smoked sausage have much more fat.

In case you haven't seen it, ancho chile pepper is found in the spice aisle along with the cayenne and Cajun seasoning. When you buy the Cajun seasoning, read the label. Get the one that has salt as low as possible on the ingredient list. This dish already has plenty of salt, so you only need the seasoning for that great Cajun pizzazz.

It's important to have all of your ingredients measured before you start cooking this recipe, or it won't be quite as easy as it really is.

1 pound boneless, skinless chicken breast, visible fat removed, cut into 2-inch cubes

3 teaspoons Cajun seasoning, divided

$1^1/_2$ tablespoons extra virgin olive oil, divided

1 large green bell pepper, cored, seeded, and coarsely chopped

2 cups coarsely chopped onion (about 1 large onion)

2 tablespoons minced fresh garlic (about 4 medium cloves)

$1^1/_2$ cups converted long-grain white rice, uncooked

$^3/_4$ pound extra-lean smoked turkey sausage or kielbasa (3 grams of fat or less per 2-ounce serving), sliced on a diagonal into $^1/_4$-inch-thick pieces

2 teaspoons dried oregano

1 tablespoon ancho chile pepper (see page 15)

Two 14.5-ounce cans no-salt-added diced tomatoes

2 large dried bay leaves

$^1/_2$ teaspoon cayenne, plus more to taste, if desired

One 14.5-ounce can fat-free or 98% fat-free, lower-sodium chicken broth (not low-sodium)

$1^1/_4$ pounds large (21–25 count) shrimp, peeled and deveined

---

MAKES ABOUT 12 CUPS; 8 SERVINGS OR 16 PORTIONS

2 Each 2-Decadent-Disk portion (about $^3/_4$ cup) has: 198 calories, 20 g protein, 20 g carbohydrates, 4 g fat, <1 g saturated fat, 84 mg cholesterol, 1 g fiber, 433 mg sodium

4 Each 4-Decadent-Disk serving (about $1^1/_2$ cups) has: 396 calories, 40 g protein, 40 g carbohydrates, 7 g fat, 2 g saturated fat, 168 mg cholesterol, 2 g fiber, 866 mg sodium

Combine the chicken and 1 teaspoon Cajun seasoning in a small bowl. Mix until the chicken is evenly coated.

Place a large nonstick saucepan over medium heat. Put in $1^1/_2$ teaspoons of the olive oil and the bell pepper, onion, and garlic. Cook, stirring occasionally, until the onion is just tender but not browning, 10 to 13 minutes. Remove the veggies and set them aside.

Turn the heat to medium-high. Put another $1^1/_2$ teaspoons of the olive oil and the rice in the pan. Cook, stirring frequently, until the rice is just starting to brown lightly, 2 to 3 minutes. Remove from the pan and transfer to a separate bowl from the veggies. Set aside.

Turn the heat to high. When the pan is hot, put in the remaining $1^1/_2$ teaspoons of olive oil. Add the chicken and cook, about 2 minutes per side, until the outsides are browned in spots. Push the chicken to the outer edges and add the sausage. Cook the sausage, stirring

occasionally, until lightly browned, 2 to 4 minutes.

Turn the heat back down to medium and add the veggies back to the pan. Add the remaining 2 teaspoons of Cajun seasoning, the oregano, and the ancho chile pepper. Stir until well combined. Cook for 5 minutes, stirring occasionally. Stir in the tomatoes, including the juice, the bay leaves, and $^1/_2$ teaspoon cayenne. Then add the chicken broth and turn the heat to high. When the liquid comes to a full boil, stir in the rice.

When it returns to a boil, turn the heat to low and cover the pan. Simmer until the rice is cooked and absorbs most of the liquid, 35 to 45 minutes.

About 5 minutes before it's cooked, stir in the shrimp and continue cooking, covered, for 5 minutes more. Remove the bay leaves. Season with cayenne to taste, if desired. Serve immediately.

HONEY-GLAZED SPICED PORK TENDERLOIN

2

I love entertaining with pork tenderloin. As long as my guests aren't averse to eating pork, it's usually one of my first choices. For years, every time I made dinner for a boyfriend's mother, I would butterfly a pork tenderloin and stuff it with goat cheese and sun-dried tomatoes. Then, in *The Biggest Loser Cookbook,* I made a Sweet and Spicy Pork Tenderloin that I started serving to guests often. I later found out that one of the producers served it to the other producers when he had them all over for dinner one night. Now here's another elegant recipe that I love, and I bet you (and your guests!) will too.

2 teaspoons paprika
$^1/_2$ teaspoon salt
1 teaspoon freshly ground black pepper
$^1/_4$ teaspoon onion powder
$^1/_8$ teaspoon chili powder
$^1/_8$ teaspoon cayenne
1$^1/_4$ pounds trimmed pork tenderloin
1 teaspoon extra virgin olive oil
1 tablespoon plus 1 teaspoon honey
1 tablespoon minced fresh garlic
Olive oil spray

Preheat the oven to 350°F.

Use a fork to mix the paprika, salt, black pepper, onion powder, chili powder, and cayenne in a small bowl.

Rub the tenderloin evenly with the olive oil. Then rub the spice mixture evenly over it until the tenderloin is thoroughly coated. Cover loosely with plastic wrap and let stand for 15 minutes.

Meanwhile, whisk the honey and garlic in a small bowl.

Place a large nonstick skillet over medium-high heat. When the skillet is hot, lightly mist it with spray. Cook the tenderloin for 1 to 2 minutes per side, or until just browned on all sides.

Place the tenderloin in a roasting pan or ovenproof skillet. (If one end is much thinner than the other, tuck it under to create a similar thickness throughout.) Use a pastry or basting brush to evenly coat the tenderloin with the honey mixture. Roast, uncovered, for 16 to 18 minutes, or until it is just barely pink inside or a meat thermometer inserted in the center reaches 155°F (the temperature will rise another 5°F while standing).

Remove from the oven, loosely cover the tenderloin (not the whole pan) with foil, and let stand for 10 minutes. Transfer the tenderloin to a cutting board. Holding your knife at a 45-degree angle, slice the tenderloin into thin slices. Serve immediately.

No more than 20 minutes hands-on prep time

MAKES 4 SERVINGS

2 Each 2-Decadent-Disk serving (about 4$^1/_2$ ounces) has: 210 calories, 30 g protein, 7 g carbohydrates, 6 g fat, 2 g saturated fat, 92 mg cholesterol, <1 g fiber, 364 mg sodium

Honey-Glazed Spiced Pork Tenderloin and Chipotle Mashed Sweet Potatoes (page 170)

MINI-MEATLOAVES

2

I've found making miniature versions of many popular dishes a great strategy for success in eating healthfully—I'm a lot less likely to dip into a second serving of something if I have to start a whole new one than I am to cut a slightly larger piece.

Here I've made these meatloaves in two mini-loaf pans that each serve 2. It's obvious where the half-way point is, so I tend to eat less. But my favorite thing to do, if you have them or can find them easily, is to bake them in four nonstick individual loaf pans (about 3 $^1/_2$ x 2 $^1/_2$ x 1 $^1/_2$ inches) instead of the two mini ones. Not only will you get to eat "the whole thing" (I find it so satisfying to finish something even if it's small), they'll definitely help keep you from "cheating" as they do for me. You'll want to bake them for only 24 to 28 minutes, though.

Olive oil spray
$^1/_3$ cup old-fashioned oats
$^1/_4$ cup fat-free milk
1 medium carrot, cut into 6 pieces
2 small whole green onions, cut in half
1 cup fresh parsley (not packed)
1 small seeded jalapeño pepper, or more to taste
1 medium garlic clove, minced
1 large egg white, lightly beaten
1 tablespoon Worcestershire sauce
1 tablespoon A.1. sauce
$^1/_3$ cup minced jarred pimientos, drained
$^1/_4$ teaspoon salt
1 pound 96% lean ground beef
$^1/_4$ cup low-sodium ketchup or ketchup, divided

Preheat the oven to 350°F.

Lightly mist 2 small (5$^3/_4$ X 3$^1/_4$-inch) nonstick loaf pans with spray.

Stir the oats into the milk in a medium mixing bowl. Let stand for 3 minutes, or until the oats are softened.

Meanwhile, put the carrot, green onions, parsley, jalapeño, and garlic in the bowl of a food processor fitted with a chopping blade. Process until minced. Transfer to a fine strainer and stir with a spoon to remove any excess moisture. Add the veggie mixture to the oat mixture. Then add the egg white, followed by the Worcestershire sauce, A.1. sauce, pimientos, and salt. Mix well. Add the beef and mix until well combined.

Divide the mixture among the prepared pans and spread it so that the tops are flat. Spread 2 tablespoons ketchup evenly over the top of each. Bake for 30 to 34 minutes, or until no longer pink inside. Remove from the oven and let stand for 10 minutes. Slice each loaf into 4 slices and serve immediately.

No more than 20 minutes hands-on prep time

MAKES 2 MINI-MEATLOAVES; 4 SERVINGS

2 Each 2-Decadent-Disk serving ($^1/_2$ loaf) has: 210 calories, 26 g protein, 15 g carbohydrates, 5 g fat, 2 g saturated fat, 60 mg cholesterol, 2 g fiber, 374 mg sodium

You save: 147 calories, 13 g fat, 3 g saturated fat

Traditional serving: 357 calories, 24 g protein, 18 g carbohydrates, 18 g fat, 5 g saturated fat, 104 mg cholesterol, <1 g fiber, 1,740 mg sodium

CHIPOTLE CHILI WITH BLUE CHEESE CRUMBLES

②

It's amazing how many versions of chili there are. I'm constantly being asked to make over people's family recipes, and no two have ever been the same.

Here is one that I particularly love that merges two of my favorite recipes. First, using the A.1. sauce to season the turkey makes the meat taste more like beef than turkey. Next, I added chipotle peppers, because chipotle was emerging as the "in thing" when I was developing the recipe. And then I topped it off with the blue cheese crumbles for a more gourmet spin. But feel free to go with the Cheddar if you're more of a traditionalist or if your favorite grocery store doesn't stock the reduced-fat blue cheese.

Look for the chipotle peppers in the international section of most grocery stores near the Mexican foods. They're pretty easy to find these days. For more info on that and the blue cheese, see pages 16 and 15.

1½ pounds extra-lean ground turkey

¼ cup A.1. sauce

Olive oil spray

1 cup chopped onions

Two 14½-ounce cans diced tomatoes

One 8-ounce can low-sodium tomato sauce

2 canned chipotle peppers in adobo sauce (about 2 tablespoons), finely chopped, or more to taste

¼ cup chili powder

1 tablespoon dark or light brown sugar

2 teaspoons Worcestershire sauce

One 15½-ounce can reduced-sodium dark kidney beans, drained

Salt and pepper

10 tablespoons crumbled reduced-fat blue cheese (or 3 ounces finely shredded Cabot's 75% Light Cheddar cheese, about 1½ cups)

Mix the turkey with the A.1. sauce in a medium bowl until just combined.

Lightly mist a large nonstick saucepan with spray and place it over medium-high heat. When the pan is hot, put in the turkey and onions. Use a wooden spoon to break the turkey into hearty chunks. Continue cooking, stirring often, until the ground turkey is no longer pink inside, 4 to 6 minutes. Add the tomatoes, tomato sauce, chipotle peppers, chili powder, brown sugar, and Worcestershire sauce. Stir until combined, then cover the pan and turn the heat to low. Simmer for at least 2 hours, stirring occasionally. Add the beans and continue cooking, uncovered, stirring occasionally until the beans are hot, about 5 minutes. Season with salt and pepper to taste. Divide the chili among 10 bowls and top each with 1 tablespoon blue cheese or 2½ tablespoons Cheddar, or refrigerate in an airtight container for up to 5 days.

No more than 20 minutes hands-on prep time

MAKES ABOUT 7½ CUPS; 10 SERVINGS

② Each 2-Decadent-Disk serving (about ¾ cup with cheese) has: 195 calories, 23 g protein, 21 g carbohydrates, 3 g fat, <1 g saturated fat, 31 mg cholesterol, 6 g fiber, 531 mg sodium

SWEET AND SLIM ITALIAN SAUSAGE

Have you ever read the label on a package of sausage? What about turkey sausage? You may be shocked to read how much fat is contained in many sausages you find in grocery stores or have ordered from restaurant menus. And my problem is that I love it.

This is one of those recipes that I developed for myself years ago because I craved sausage. You'll notice that I use actual ground pork in this recipe. With only about 3.5 grams of fat for 4 ounces, there's no reason not to use it. I flavor the pork with the seasonings used in traditional sweet Italian sausage and create a similar texture by adding moisture with the combo of bread crumbs and egg substitute.

I wouldn't trade this for the world. True, it contains more salt than I'd like, but I did cut as much as I could without sacrificing that authentic taste. In the end, it has even 44 fewer calories and 7 fewer grams of fat than the leanest chicken or turkey sausage found in my local grocery store, and way less than that as compared to real pork sausage.

Olive oil spray (must use real olive oil not Pam)

1 pound extra-lean ground pork or pork tenderloin, ground

$^1/_4$ cup plus 1 tablespoon egg substitute

$^1/_4$ cup plus 1 tablespoon plain dried bread crumbs

1 tablespoon plus 1 teaspoon fennel seeds

$1^1/_2$ teaspoons garlic powder

1 teaspoon Italian seasoning

1 teaspoon onion powder

$^3/_4$ teaspoon salt

$^1/_2$ teaspoon cayenne

$^1/_2$ teaspoon black pepper

Preheat the oven to 400°F.

Lightly mist a small nonstick baking sheet with spray.

Mix the pork, egg substitute, bread crumbs, fennel seeds, garlic powder, Italian seasoning, onion powder, salt, cayenne, and black pepper in a medium mixing bowl. Divide into 8 equal amounts (about a heaping $^1/_4$ cup each). Shape each into a log about 4 inches long and $1^1/_2$ inches thick. Place the logs side by side, not touching, on the prepared baking sheet. Mist them lightly with spray. Bake for 9 to 11 minutes, until no longer pink inside. Serve immediately.

Can be made in 30 minutes or less / No more than 20 minutes hands-on prep time

MAKES 8 LINKS; 8 SERVINGS

Each 1-Decadent-Disk portion (1 link) has: 96 calories, 14 g protein, 4 g carbohydrates, 2 g fat, <1 g saturated fat, 37 mg cholesterol, <1 g fiber, 293 mg sodium

You save: 184 calories, 22 g fat, 7 g saturated fat

Traditional serving (1 link): 280 calories, 12 g protein, 3 g carbohydrates, 24 g fat, 8 g saturated fat, 55 mg cholesterol, trace fiber, 980 mg sodium

LEMON-THYME CHICKEN KEBABS

2

When I first made these chicken kebabs, I wasn't so sure how I felt about them. I knew they were tasty, but I wondered if they had a wow-factor worthy of *The Most Decadent Diet Ever!* So I served them at a taste-testing party, and they were a hit. My friend Jen even begged me for the recipe right on the spot; she went home and made them twice within the next few days.

Whatever you do, don't use bottled lemon juice. I never actually recommend doing that, but sometimes, when you're using just a little bit, it's not a big deal. The lemon flavor is too pronounced here—the result might not be to your liking.

If you're using wooden skewers, be sure to soak them for at least $1/2$ hour (up to a day before) so they don't burn on the grill. The metal ones obviously don't need to be soaked.

$1/3$ cup fresh lemon juice
2 tablespoons minced fresh garlic
2 tablespoons finely chopped fresh thyme
1 tablespoon plus 1 teaspoon extra virgin olive oil
2 teaspoons honey
$1/2$ teaspoon salt

$1^1/4$ pounds boneless, skinless chicken breasts, visible fat removed
$1/2$ cup 1-inch red onion squares (20 to 25 pieces)
4 metal or wooden skewers soaked in water for at least 30 minutes

Whisk the lemon juice, garlic, thyme, olive oil, honey, and salt in a small bowl.

Cut the chicken into $1^1/2$-inch cubes. Transfer the cubes to a resealable container and pour the marinade over the top. Toss the chicken in the marinade. Seal the container and refrigerate for at least 6 hours or overnight, rotating it at least once.

Preheat a grill to high.

Place a piece of onion on a skewer. Add a cube of chicken, then another piece of onion. Repeat, dividing the chicken among 4 skewers, beginning and ending with onion on each. Discard any remaining marinade.

Place the kebabs side by side on the grill. Turn the heat to medium, if possible. Cook for 2 minutes, rotate $1/4$ turn, and cook for another 1 to 2 minutes per side, until the chicken is no longer pink inside. Serve immediately.

MAKES 4 KEBABS; 4 SERVINGS

2 Each 2-Decadent-Disk serving (1 kebab) has: 197 calories, 33 g protein, 5 g carbohydrates, 4 g fat, <1 g saturated fat, 82 mg cholesterol, <1 g fiber, 239 mg sodium

You save: 187 calories, 22 g fat, 3 g saturated fat

Traditional serving: 384 calories, 31 g protein, 5 g carbohydrates, 26 g fat, 4 g saturated fat, 82 mg cholesterol, trace fiber, 656 mg sodium

GRILLED CHICKEN QUESADILLA

In Mexican dishes, chicken is often shredded. I like hearty bites of chicken, so I grill mine. I like the consistency better, and I don't need a fatty simmering liquid to yield tender chicken. With leftover grilled chicken, this is a cinch to make, and it's a kid-pleaser too (you might want to hold back on the seasoning and jalapeños if you're serving this to little ones).

Feel free to add more salsa here (I love the fresh over jarred varieties). With only 5 calories per tablespoon, you really can't go wrong.

Please be sure to wash your hands after working with jalapeños. My friend John touched his eyes after making one of my recipes with jalapeños. I got an e-mail saying, "Great lobster cakes, you owe me an eye patch." Fortunately, his eye was just slightly irritated, but it can be painful, so be careful.

1 teaspoon salt-free Mexican or Southwest seasoning (see page 17)
$^1/_4$ teaspoon onion powder
Pinch of garlic powder
Pinch of salt
One 3-ounce boneless, skinless chicken breast, visible fat removed
1 (about 8-inch diameter) low-fat, whole-wheat flour tortilla

$1^1/_2$ ounces ($^3/_4$ cup) finely shredded Cabot's 75% Light Cheddar cheese, or your favorite low-fat Cheddar
1 tablespoon finely chopped whole green onion
1 teaspoon finely chopped fresh cilantro
1 teaspoon seeded and minced green jalapeño pepper, or more to taste
1 to 2 tablespoons fresh salsa

Preheat the oven to 350°F.

Preheat a grill to high.

Mix the Mexican seasoning, onion powder, garlic powder, and salt in a small bowl. Rub the mixture evenly over the chicken. Let stand for 10 minutes.

Place the chicken on the grill and turn the heat to medium, if possible. Grill for 2 to 4 minutes per side, or until no longer pink inside. Let stand for 5 to 10 minutes, until cooled, and then coarsely chop it.

Place the tortilla on a nonstick baking sheet. Sprinkle half of the cheese evenly over half of the tortilla, followed by the chicken, green onion, cilantro, jalapeño, and finally the remaining cheese. Fold the bare half over the filling. Bake for 4 to 7 minutes, or until the cheese is melted.

Use a spatula to transfer the quesadilla to a clean, dry cutting board. Slice it into 4 wedges. Then transfer the wedges to a plate and top with salsa to taste. Serve immediately.

No more than 20 minutes hands-on prep time

MAKES 1 QUESADILLA; 1 SERVING

Each 3-Decadent-Disk serving (1 quesadilla) has: 303 calories, 36 g protein, 26 g carbohydrates, 7 g fat, 3 g saturated fat, 65 mg cholesterol, 2 g fiber, 650 mg sodium

You save: 172 calories, 20 g fat, 11 g saturated fat

Traditional serving: 475 calories, 30 g protein, 29 g carbohydrates, 27 g fat, 14 g saturated fat, 98 mg cholesterol, 2 g fiber, 980 mg sodium

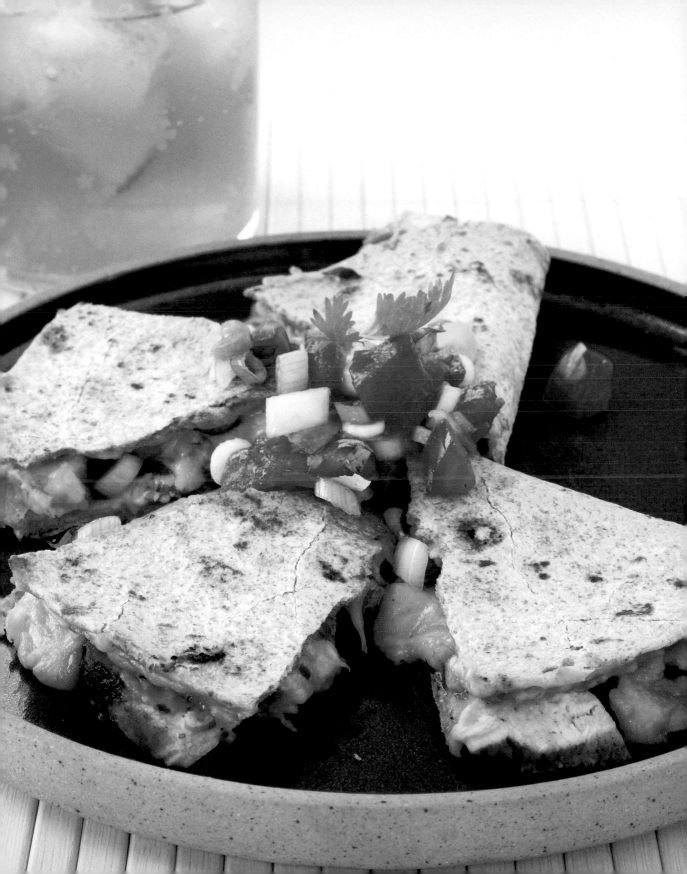

CHICKEN ENCHILASAGNA

2 **4**

I'd gotten so many requests from fans to make over enchiladas that I started playing around with the ingredients to see what I could do. After perfecting them, I decided I needed to figure out a way to cut the prep time. And so, this recipe was born. This is as easy as making a throw-together lasagna. Plus, it's nice and lean with a great protein-to-carbohydrate ratio, and it tastes just as decadent as restaurant enchiladas.

2 teaspoons salt-free Mexican or Southwest seasoning (see page 17)
2 teaspoons lower-sodium burrito seasoning or taco seasoning (see pages 15 and 18)
1¼ pounds boneless, skinless chicken breasts, visible fat removed
Olive oil spray
1¼ cups canned traditional mild enchilada sauce
1 cup canned medium green chile enchilada sauce
4 ounces (about 2 cups) finely shredded Cabot's 75% Light Cheddar cheese, or your favorite low-fat Cheddar
½ cup chopped fresh cilantro
¼ cup sliced drained black olives
3 tablespoons canned, drained, and chopped green chiles
Eight 6-inch white or yellow corn tortillas

Preheat a grill to high.
Preheat the oven to 450°F.
Mix the Mexican seasoning and burrito seasoning in a small bowl. Rub the mixture evenly over the chicken breasts to cover them. Lightly mist both sides of the breasts with spray. Let stand for 10 minutes, and then place the breasts side by side on the grill. Turn the heat to medium, if possible, and grill for 3 to 5 minutes per side, or until no longer pink inside. Let stand for 5 minutes.

Meanwhile, combine the enchilada sauces in a medium bowl and mix until well combined. Set aside.

Mix the cheese, cilantro, olives, and chiles in a second medium bowl. Set aside.

Coarsely chop the chicken breasts.

Cut or tear each tortilla into about 9 roughly even pieces.

Spread ½ cup of the enchilada sauce in the bottom of an 8 X 8-inch glass or ceramic baking dish. Cover the sauce evenly with about a third of the tortilla pieces. Then sprinkle about half of the chicken over them. Pour about ⅔ cup of the sauce evenly over that. Then sprinkle a third of the cheese mixture over that.

Repeat layering with half of the remaining tortillas, the remaining chicken, ⅔ cup of sauce, then half of the remaining cheese mixture. Follow that with another layer of the tortillas, then the remaining sauce, then the remaining cheese mixture. Cover with foil and bake for 25 minutes. Remove the foil and bake for another 5 minutes. Then remove from the oven and let stand for 10 minutes. Cut into 4 or 8 pieces and serve immediately.

MAKES 1 CASSEROLE; 4 SERVINGS OR 8 PORTIONS

2 Each 2-Decadent-Disk portion (⅛ casserole) has: 201 calories, 23 g protein, 16 g carbohydrates, 5 g fat, 1 g saturated fat, 46 mg cholesterol, 2 g fiber, 531 mg sodium

4 Each 4-Decadent-Disk serving (¼ casserole) has: 401 calories, 46 g protein, 32 g carbohydrates, 9 g fat, 2 g saturated fat, 92 mg cholesterol, 4 g fiber, 1,063 mg sodium

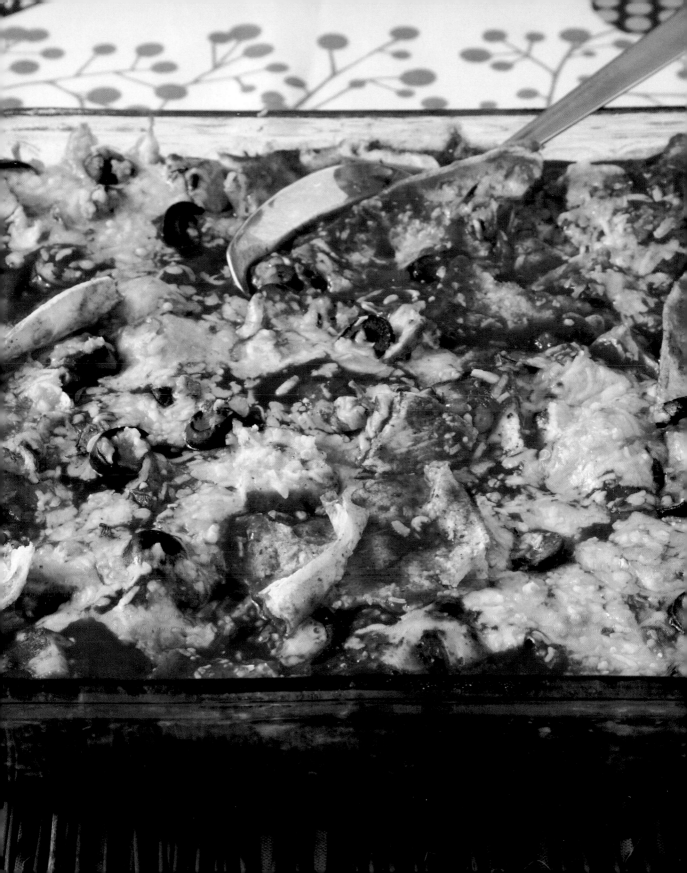

CHICKEN PICCATA

2

When I moved to Los Angeles, I happened upon a guy from Boston who always hosted Sunday dinners. Mike would gather his friends from the East Coast every Sunday night and make an Italian Sunday dinner just like his family did back in Boston. I managed to get myself invited and, in my early days in L.A., it was probably the outing I most looked forward to each week.

After a couple of years, Mike got too busy with his job at Sony to keep them going. So I started hosting them. At first, they were simply a way to gather friends. But they later turned into a great vehicle to test new recipes.

I'm not in town enough these days to host them as often as I'd like. But I do still host a Sunday dinner when I have new recipes I want to try out on an audience. And since these dinners are so casual, everyone feels comfortable telling the truth as to whether they love the recipes. This recipe received very high praise.

It's very important to have your ingredients premeasured for this dish before you actually start cooking. If you don't, the sauce could pose a challenge. Otherwise, it's a cinch!

$2\frac{1}{2}$ tablespoons unbleached all-purpose flour, divided
$\frac{1}{4}$ teaspoon salt, plus more to taste
$\frac{1}{4}$ teaspoon black pepper, plus more to taste
$\frac{1}{4}$ teaspoon garlic powder
Four 4-ounce boneless, skinless chicken breasts, visible fat removed
$\frac{1}{4}$ cup fat-free half-and-half
2 teaspoons plus 2 tablespoons light butter (stick, not tub), divided, room temperature
$\frac{1}{2}$ cup canned fat-free, lower-sodium chicken broth, plus more if needed
$\frac{1}{3}$ cup dry white wine
$\frac{1}{4}$ cup fresh lemon juice
$1\frac{1}{2}$ teaspoons minced fresh garlic
2 tablespoons capers, drained
2 tablespoons chopped fresh parsley

Combine $1\frac{1}{2}$ tablespoons of the flour with $\frac{1}{4}$ teaspoon salt, $\frac{1}{4}$ teaspoon pepper, and the garlic powder on a dinner plate. Use a fork or your fingers to mix well.

Pat the chicken breasts dry with paper towels to ensure that they are as dry as possible. Place them between two sheets of plastic wrap or wax paper on a flat work

---

MAKES 4 SERVINGS

2 Each 2-Decadent-Disk serving (1 chicken breast with 2 to $2\frac{1}{2}$ tablespoons sauce) has: 206 calories, 28 g protein, 8 g carbohydrates, 5 g fat, 3 g saturated fat, 77 mg cholesterol, trace fiber, 469 mg sodium

You save: 71 calories, 11 g fat, 5 g saturated fat

Traditional serving: 277 calories, 26 g protein, 8 g carbohydrates, 16 g fat, 8 g saturated fat, 146 mg cholesterol, <1 g fiber, 574 mg sodium

surface. Use the flat side of a meat mallet to pound them to an even $^1/_4$-inch thickness. Dip one breast at a time into the flour mixture to coat on all sides. Shake off any excess and transfer the breasts, to a clean plate, side by side (don't pile them on top of each other).

Put the remaining 1 tablespoon of flour in a small, deep bowl. Whisk in enough half-and-half to form a paste. Then continue whisking in the remaining half-and-half until well combined. Set aside.

Place a large nonstick skillet over high heat. When the skillet is hot, put in 2 teaspoons butter. Spread it to cover the bottom of the skillet and immediately add the chicken breasts, side by side. Cook until golden brown on both sides and no longer pink inside (if they're browning too much, turn the heat

down), about 3 minutes per side. Transfer the chicken to a platter and tent it with foil to keep warm.

Add the chicken broth, wine, lemon juice, and garlic to the skillet. When the liquid is reduced by half, 1 to 2 minutes (the alcohol should be burned off), turn the heat to low. Whisk in the half-and-half mixture until well combined. Add the remaining 2 tablespoons butter. Continue whisking until the mixture is smooth and the butter is completely melted. If the sauce is too thin, continue whisking until it thickens slightly. If it's too thick, add more chicken broth, 1 tablespoon at a time, until it reaches the consistency of a gravy. Stir in the capers. Season with salt and pepper to taste. Spoon the sauce evenly over the chicken. Garnish with parsley and serve immediately.

CHICKEN CORDON BLEU

3

I think chicken cordon bleu must be the official banquet entrée of Pennsylvania (at least in Reading, the part of Pennsylvania where I grew up). Whether it was my brother's sports banquet or our church fund-raising banquet that I was being dragged to, I knew I'd be eating it. I truly don't remember ever being to a banquet where it wasn't served.

Since I loved fried food, I was never disappointed. But imagine my surprise when I moved to Los Angeles and people barely knew what it was—they certainly weren't eating it or serving it en masse. It's probably a good thing it's not served countrywide, especially when you consider the fat and calories of the traditional version.

I developed this recipe using 97% lean ham, even though I recently happened upon 99%, which was equally tasty—I was afraid folks might not be able to find the 99% lean easily. If you can, definitely use that. You'll save even more fat and calories.

Note that you can stuff and bread the chicken up to one day in advance for convenience. Then bake it just before eating.

Olive oil spray (real olive oil; not Pam)
3 tablespoons unbleached all-purpose flour
$1/4$ teaspoon salt, plus more to taste
$1/4$ teaspoon black pepper, plus more to taste
$1/4$ teaspoon garlic powder
$1/8$ teaspoon paprika
2 large egg whites
1 tablespoon fat-free milk
$1/2$ cup dried bread crumbs
$1^1/2$ teaspoons finely chopped fresh parsley
Four 5-ounce boneless, skinless chicken breasts, visible fat removed
3 ounces sliced 97% lean deli ham
$3^1/2$ ounces light Swiss cheese slivers

Preheat the oven to 450°F.

Lightly mist a medium nonstick baking sheet with spray.

Arrange 3 medium shallow bowls side by side. Mix the flour, $1/4$ teaspoon salt, and $1/4$ teaspoon pepper with the garlic powder and paprika in the first bowl. Use a fork to lightly beat the egg whites with the milk in the second bowl. Mix the bread crumbs and the parsley in the third bowl.

Pat the chicken breasts dry with paper

MAKES 4 SERVINGS

3 Each 3-Decadent-Disk serving (1 chicken breast) has: 306 calories, 48 g protein, 10 g carbohydrates, 7 g fat, 2 g saturated fat, 101 mg cholesterol, <1 g fiber, 599 mg sodium

You save: 215 calories, 24 g fat

Traditional serving: 521 calories, 47 g protein, 12 g carbohydrates, 31 g fat, saturated fat N/A, cholesterol N/A, <1 g fiber, sodium N/A

towels to ensure that they are as dry as possible. Place them between two sheets of plastic wrap or wax paper on a flat work surface. Use the flat side of a meat mallet to pound them to an even $^1/_8$- to $^1/_4$-inch thickness. Then place them on the wrap or paper with the top of the breasts facedown and season with salt and pepper to taste.

Place a quarter of the ham and then a quarter of the cheese evenly in the center of each breast, about $^1/_2$ inch from each edge. Roll the breasts lengthwise so the seams end up on the bottom. If desired, fasten the breasts with toothpicks inserted near the bottom so that the breasts remain rolled.

Next, being careful not to unroll it, dip one of the breasts into the flour mixture until it is coated on all sides. Shake off any excess flour, and then dip it into the egg mixture. Allow any excess egg to drip from the chicken, and then coat it with bread crumbs. Place seam side down on the prepared baking sheet, making sure to tuck the sides under slightly.

Prepare the 3 remaining chicken breasts following the same procedure, placing them side by side, not touching, on the prepared baking sheet. Lightly mist the tops with spray. Bake for approximately 9 minutes. Then carefully flip the breasts over (using tongs is easiest) and bake for another 9 to 12 minutes, or until no longer pink inside. Serve immediately.

GRILLED CHICKEN WITH BRUSCHETTA TOPPING

2

You've probably been to plenty of parties where bruschetta has been served. It's that crisped bread with the wonderfully garlicky fresh tomatoes on top. Well, here's a twist on that. It makes for a super-lean meal full of great muscle-building protein and cancer-preventing tomatoes, with tons of flavor and only heart-healthy fats. It's particularly great for a summer day when fresh tomatoes are in season and thus tend to be less expensive and even more delicious.

1 recipe Bruschetta Topping (recipe follows)
Four 4^1/2-ounce boneless, skinless chicken
    breasts, visible fat removed
1 teaspoon extra virgin olive oil
1^1/2 teaspoons minced fresh garlic
Salt and pepper

Prepare the Bruschetta Topping.
    Preheat a grill to high.
    Place the chicken breasts between two sheets of plastic wrap or wax paper on a flat work surface. Use the flat side of a meat mallet to pound them to an even ^{1}/2-inch thickness.
    Transfer the chicken to a medium bowl. Add the olive oil and garlic. Mix with your hands until well combined. Season generously with salt and pepper to taste.
    Place the chicken breasts side by side on the grill. Turn the heat to medium, if possible, and grill for 3 to 5 minutes per side, until no longer pink inside. Transfer to a platter or individual plates and spoon a quarter of the Bruschetta Topping (about ^{1}/4 cup) over each. Serve immediately.

BRUSCHETTA TOPPING

1^1/3 cups seeded and finely chopped Roma
    tomatoes (see page 21)
1 tablespoon finely slivered fresh basil leaves (see
    page 20)
1 tablespoon extra virgin olive oil
1^1/2 teaspoons balsamic vinegar
1 teaspoon minced or crushed fresh garlic
^{1}/2 teaspoon sugar
^{1}/4 teaspoon salt
Pinch of black pepper, or to taste

Mix the tomatoes, basil, olive oil, vinegar, garlic, sugar, salt, and pepper in a medium resealable container. Seal the container and refrigerate for at least 2 hours to let the flavors meld. Serve cold or at room temperature.

Makes 1 to 1^1/4 cups; 8 servings
Each 2-tablespoon serving has: 23 calories, <1 g protein, 2 g carbohydrates, 2 g fat, <1 g saturated fat, 0 mg cholesterol, <1 g fiber, 75 mg sodium

---

MAKES 4 SERVINGS

2 Each 2-Decadent-Disk serving (1 chicken breast plus ^{1}/4 recipe Bruschetta Topping) has:
199 calories, 30 g protein, 4 g carbohydrates, 6 g fat, 1 g saturated fat, 74 mg cholesterol, <1 g fiber, 232 mg sodium

POTATO CHIP-CRUSTED CHICKEN

✹ **2**

People often ask how I come up with my recipes, and I often say, "Trial and error and error and error." And it's true. Sometimes I get lucky and a dish comes together immediately. But more often, it takes attempt after attempt to get a recipe right. This dish is an example. I set out to make the recipes in this book defy the label "diet food." I wanted you to be able to flip through the book and say, "How could that be healthy?" and then dig in and realize that healthier food can actually taste great.

As I was reading a magazine one day, I saw a version of potato chip chicken where they dipped the whole chicken parts with the skin still on in butter, then in tons of crushed full-fat potato chips. Yikes! But I thought it was an interesting, definitely decadent-sounding idea. So I set out to coat the chicken in Baked! Ruffles. The first attempt was really bland. We decided that perhaps the sour cream and cheddar ones would work better. But they didn't. Then we tried Doritos-crusted chicken, thinking that the strong nacho cheese flavor would give it the right zip. Wrong again. Finally, after many spice variations, I arrived at this version using the baked Ruffles one afternoon. My computer consultant, Corbin, happened to be working on my computer that day (he loves food and his mom is a chef), so I had him try it. He was a huge fan, and a recipe was born.

It's really easy to crush the chips if you put them in a resealable plastic bag and pound them with the flat side of a meat mallet or a rolling pin. They should be pretty finely crushed or you won't be able to coat the breasts completely.

Two 3-ounce boneless, skinless chicken breasts, visible fat removed
$1/3$ cup low-fat buttermilk
Olive oil spray
$1/2$ teaspoon onion powder
$1/4$ teaspoon paprika
$1/4$ teaspoon black pepper
$1/8$ teaspoon salt
Pinch of cayenne
$1 1/2$ ounces (about $1/2$ cup) finely crushed Baked! Ruffles potato chips

Place the chicken breasts between two sheets of plastic wrap or wax paper on a flat work surface. Use the flat side of a meat mallet to pound them to an even $1/2$-inch thickness. Put the chicken breasts in a resealable plastic bag that is slightly larger than the breasts. Pour the buttermilk over the breasts, seal the bag, and then turn the bag to coat. Refrigerate for at least 6 hours or overnight, rotating once or twice.

Preheat the oven to 450°F.   *(continued)*

Can be made in 30 minutes or less / No more than 20 minutes hands-on prep time

---

MAKES 2 SERVINGS

✹**2** Each 2-Decadent-Disk (1 chicken breast) serving has: 206 calories, 22 g protein, 20 g carbohydrates, 4 g fat, trace saturated fat, 51 mg cholesterol, <1 g fiber, 376 mg sodium

Lightly mist a small nonstick baking sheet with spray.

Mix the onion powder, paprika, black pepper, salt, and cayenne in a small bowl.

Put the chips in a medium shallow bowl.

Remove one chicken breast from the buttermilk and let any excess buttermilk drip off. Sprinkle both sides of the breast evenly with half of the seasoning mixture. Then transfer the breast to the bowl of crushed chips and cover completely with the chips.

Place the coated breast on the prepared baking sheet. Repeat with the remaining chicken breast. Discard any remaining marinade.

Lightly mist the top of both breasts with spray. Bake for 4 minutes, and then carefully flip the breasts with a spatula, being sure not the remove the coating. Lightly mist the tops with spray and bake for another 3 to 5 minutes, or until the coating is crispy and the chicken is no longer pink inside. Serve immediately.

Potato Chip–Crusted Chicken with Grilled Corn on the Cob (page 182)

GENERAL PAO'S CHICKEN

2

You may be thinking, "Isn't it General Tso's Chicken?" Well, at your favorite local Chinese restaurant, I bet it is. But this dish is something I put together one night when I was craving Chinese food. It isn't a dead-on re-creation of any actual Chinese food dish, but it is, arguably, a cross between the traditional General Tso's and kung pao chicken … with a lot less fat, fewer calories, and much less sodium. So if you're a fan of either of those dishes, you're likely to love this one too. It's great served with brown rice or whole-grain pilaf.

Just be sure that when you cook the chicken, the pan is nice and hot and the chicken stays in a single layer. You really want the chicken to at least lightly brown on the outsides before cooking all of the way through to achieve a true Chinese restaurant–quality result. And when you buy the hoisin sauce, if your grocery store carries more than one brand, buy the one with the least sodium. They vary widely and this dish doesn't need the extra found in some brands.

1$\frac{1}{4}$ pounds boneless, skinless chicken breasts, visible fat removed

3 tablespoons cornstarch, divided

$\frac{1}{3}$ cup 98% fat-free or fat-free, lower-sodium chicken broth

3 tablespoons lower-sodium soy sauce

2 tablespoons rice vinegar

1$\frac{1}{2}$ tablespoons sugar

1 tablespoon sherry

1$\frac{1}{2}$ teaspoons hoisin sauce

1$\frac{1}{2}$ teaspoons minced peeled fresh ginger

1$\frac{1}{2}$ teaspoons minced fresh garlic

1 teaspoon finely chopped dried red chiles, or to taste

2 teaspoons toasted sesame oil, divided

1 medium red bell pepper, cut into 1-inch pieces

1 cup 1-inch onion squares

$\frac{1}{3}$ cup chopped whole green onions

Can be made in 30 minutes or less

MAKES ABOUT 5 CUPS; 5 SERVINGS

2 Each 2-Decadent-Disk serving (scant 1 cup) has: 206 calories, 28 g protein, 15 g carbohydrates, 3 g fat, <1 g saturated fat, 66 mg cholesterol, 1 g fiber, 480 mg sodium

You save: 261 calories, 27 g fat, 5 g saturated fat

Traditional serving: 467 calories, 32 g protein, 17 g carbohydrates, 30 g fat, 6 g saturated fat, 72 mg cholesterol, 4 g fiber, 591 mg sodium

Place the chicken breasts between two sheets of plastic wrap or wax paper on a flat work surface. Use the flat side of a meat mallet to pound them to an even $1/3$-inch thickness. Cut the breasts into $3/4$-inch strips. Transfer to a medium bowl and add 2 tablespoons cornstarch. Toss to coat well. Let stand for 5 minutes.

Meanwhile, whisk the remaining cornstarch and the broth, soy sauce, vinegar, sugar, sherry, hoisin sauce, ginger, garlic, and chiles in a medium bowl until the sugar is dissolved and the mixture is well combined.

Place a large nonstick wok or stir-fry pan over high heat. When the wok is hot, put in 1 teaspoon sesame oil. Add the bell pepper and white onions. Cook, stirring frequently, until the veggies are crisp-tender, but not yet browned, 3 to 5 minutes. Remove them from the wok and set aside.

Put in the remaining teaspoon of sesame oil and the chicken in a single layer. When the chicken is lightly browned on one side, after about 2 minutes, flip it and let the other side brown lightly. Then continue cooking, stirring occasionally, until no longer pink inside. Return the bell pepper and onions to the pan, and then add the sauce. Use a wooden spoon to stir the mixture constantly until the sauce thickens just enough to stick to the chicken and a little bit remains in the wok. Transfer the chicken and vegetables to a serving platter and top with the green onions. Serve immediately.

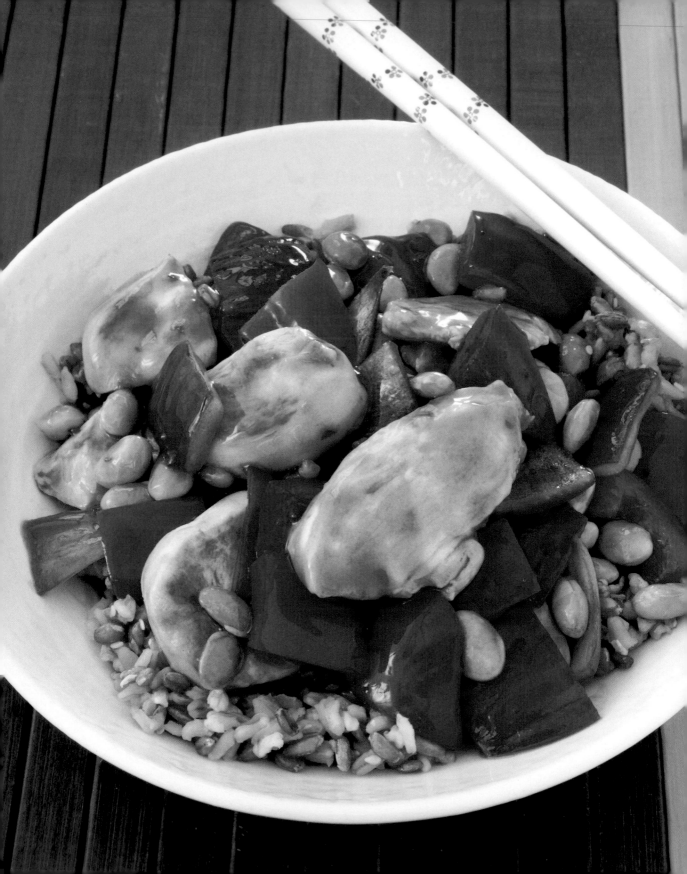

SWEET-AND-SOUR CHICKEN BOWL

5

I used to be nearly addicted to those fast-food-type Chinese restaurants in the food courts at malls. All of those bowls were just so tasty, but so bad for me.

The sweet-and-sour chicken bowl was definitely one of my all-time favorites. I loved the fried morsels of chicken nestled in lots of gooey sweet sauce, served over white rice, but my body certainly did not. There really isn't much nutritional value in a pile of overly breaded and fried dark-meat chicken.

Note that this is the highest-calorie dish in the book, and the serving size is not huge. That said, it's a full meal, inclusive of lean meat and soy protein, veggies, and a full 10 grams of fiber. As decadent as it tastes, you'd never guess it packs all of those nutrients.

2 tablespoons frozen shelled soybeans (edamame)

1 teaspoon cornstarch

$1/4$ teaspoon garlic powder

$1/8$ teaspoon salt

Black pepper

Pinch of cayenne

One 4-ounce boneless, skinless chicken breast, visible fat removed, cut diagonally across the breast into 7 or 8 equal strips

1 teaspoon toasted sesame oil

$1/4$ cup $3/4$-inch red bell pepper squares

$1/4$ cup $3/4$-inch red onion squares

$1^1/2$ teaspoons minced fresh garlic

1 tablespoon plus 2 teaspoons bottled sweet-and-sour stir-fry sauce (or sweet-and-sour sauce), divided

$2/3$ cup cooked whole-grain pilaf (such as Kashi seven-whole-grain pilaf; see page 17), reheated if necessary

Bring 2 cups salted water to a boil in a small saucepan. Add the soybeans. Cook for 5 minutes, and then drain well.

Meanwhile, mix the cornstarch, garlic powder, salt, pepper to taste, and cayenne in a medium bowl until combined. Add the chicken and toss until evenly coated.

Place a medium nonstick wok or skillet over high heat. When the wok is hot, put in the sesame oil. Add the soybeans, bell pepper, onion, and garlic. Cook until the garlic begins to soften, 1 to 2 minutes. Push the veggies to the outer edges of the pan.

Add the chicken in a single layer in the center. Cook the chicken until it is lightly browned on the bottom. Flip the chicken to cook the other side. Stir the veggies, still keeping them at the edges of the pan. When the chicken is browned, stir the chicken and veggies together and continue cooking, stirring constantly, until the chicken is no longer pink inside and the veggies are crisp-tender. Turn the heat off and add 1 tablespoon sweet-and-sour sauce. Mix well.

Spoon the pilaf into the bottom of a medium shallow bowl and level it to create an even layer. Drizzle the remaining 2 teaspoons sauce evenly over the pilaf. Mound the chicken mixture over the pilaf. Serve immediately.

MAKES 1 SERVING

5 Each 5-Decadent-Disk serving (1 bowl) has: 500 calories, 38 g protein, 61 g carbohydrates, 11 g fat, 1 g saturated fat, 66 mg cholesterol, 10 g fiber, 413 mg sodium

SAGE BUTTER ROASTED TURKEY WITH MADEIRA WINE GRAVY

2

If you've never used an oven bag to roast turkey, you're missing out. They enable you to take a lean breast, remove the skin, and still achieve an incredibly tender result. This recipe is a great candidate for a first-time effort: it takes only minutes to get the breast in the oven and you'll have a scrumptious meal, with plenty of leftovers. The leftovers are great for turkey sandwiches like Turkey Sandwich with Cranberry Aioli (page 66) and keep you from running to the local deli. Not only will the turkey be fresh, you'll save money over buying it precooked, and it will have a lot less sodium than most store-bought varieties.

Four ounces of this cooked turkey will have about 257 milligrams of sodium. Most "lower-sodium" turkey breast typically has as many as 720 milligrams per 4-ounce serving. Seasoned varieties of deli-bought turkey are likely to have about 880 milligrams of sodium.

You'll notice that I instruct you to poke the turkey with a fork. This is another technique you can use when cooking any turkey breast. It helps the seasonings seep into the breast and eliminates the need for marinating.

If you enjoy turkey without the gravy, feel free to skip it and serve the turkey with the drippings. You'll save 31 calories and 1 gram of fat per serving.

One 3-pound, bone-in turkey breast half
2 tablespoons light butter (stick, not tub), room temperature
1 tablespoon finely chopped fresh sage
$^1/_2$ teaspoon salt
$^1/_8$ teaspoon freshly ground black pepper
1 tablespoon unbleached all-purpose flour
$^3/_4$ cup plus 2 tablespoons Madeira Wine Gravy (recipe follows)

Preheat the oven to 325°F.

Place the turkey breast on a cutting board. Remove the skin. Use a fork to poke the breast 25 times, as deep as the tines of the fork, evenly covering both sides of the breast.

Mix the butter, sage, salt, and pepper in a small bowl until well combined. Rub the butter mixture over the breast, but not over the ribs (it will not melt in), spreading it as evenly as possible over both sides and the top of the breast.

Put the flour in a small oven roasting bag and shake the bag (the flour prevents the bag from popping). Put the bag in a medium roasting pan, and then place the breast, rib side down, in the bag. Insert a meat thermometer in the thickest part of the breast so it does not hit a bone. Loosely tie the bag so that the top does not touch the top of the breast.

No more than 20 minutes hands-on prep time

MAKES 7 SERVINGS

2 Each 2-Decadent-Disk serving (about 4 ounces turkey plus 2 tablespoons gravy) has: 205 calories, 34 g protein, 3 g carbohydrates, 4 g fat, 2 g saturated fat, 105 mg cholesterol, trace fiber, 336 mg sodium

Roast the breast for 1 hour to 1 hour and 10 minutes, or until the thermometer reads 175°F (the temperature will rise another 5°F while standing) and the breast is no longer pink inside.

Remove from the oven and let stand in the bag for 10 minutes. Carefully, so that the turkey drippings remain in the bag (the drippings will be used), open the bag. Remove the breast from the bag and transfer it to a cutting board. Spoon the drippings from the bag into a bowl. Slice the turkey against the grain. (If using leftovers as deli meat, slice only the portion you are eating, then refrigerate the remainder in an airtight container and slice it as thinly as possible just before eating). Serve one seventh of the turkey (about 4 ounces) with 2 tablespoons of gravy or drippings over the top.

MADEIRA WINE GRAVY

When making Sage Butter Roasted Turkey it's great to use the drippings from the turkey in place of some of the broth here (you're not likely to have a full 1/2 cups) Not only will it add a richness, you'll save even more sodium. But whether it's made with drippings or broth, you're bound to want to use this gravy on mashed potatoes, on stuffing, and even with biscuits. With only 31 calories and 1 gram of fat for a 2-tablespoon serving, you really can't go wrong.

2 tablespoons unbleached all-purpose flour
1^1/2 cups low-fat, lower-sodium turkey stock or chicken broth and/or turkey drippings from Sage Butter Roasted Turkey (page 148)
^{1}/2 cup Madeira wine
2 tablespoons light butter (stick, not tub)

Spoon the flour into a medium mixing bowl. Whisk in enough broth to form a paste. Continue whisking in the broth until well combined and no lumps remain. Set aside.

Place a medium saucepan over medium-high heat. Put in the Madeira and the broth mixture. Bring the mixture to a boil and reduce the heat to medium. Whisk the mixture occasionally until it thickens to the consistency of gravy, 4 to 6 minutes. Whisk in the butter until melted and well combined.

Makes about 1^1/4 cups; 11 servings
Each 2-tablespoon serving has: 31 calories, <1 g protein, 5 g carbohydrates, 1 g fat, 1 g saturated fat, 3 mg cholesterol, <1 g fiber, 80 mg sodium

PAN-"FRIED" SALMON WITH MANGO CUCUMBER SALSA

2

Salsas are one of my all-time favorite healthy foods because they have so much flavor for so few calories. Because the ingredients are cut so finely, the veggies (or the fruit, in some salsas) provide a flavor explosion in your mouth. Thus you don't need to add a lot of fats or oils to have a wonderfully indulgent meal.

When buying salmon, always get the thickest pieces possible. Pieces closer to the head are always better; because the tail does the work to help the fish swim, the tail end is tougher. If you go to buy fish and they have whole fillets, ask them to cut "the top half." More often than not, they'll do it for you and you'll get the best piece to cut into smaller pieces.

$1/4$ teaspoon ground cumin
$1/8$ teaspoon salt, plus more to taste
Pinch of cayenne, plus more to taste, if desired
Two 4-ounce salmon fillets, skin and bones removed
Olive oil spray
Black pepper (optional)
$1/2$ cup plus 2 tablespoons Mango Cucumber Salsa (recipe follows)

Mix the cumin, $1/8$ teaspoon salt, and pinch of cayenne in a small bowl until combined.

Lightly mist both sides of the salmon fillets with spray. Sprinkle the spice mixture evenly over both sides.

Place a small nonstick skillet over medium-high heat. When the pan is hot, put in the fillets.

Cook until the outsides are just lightly browned, 1 to 2 minutes per side. Then turn the heat to medium and cook until the salmon is a pale pink throughout, 2 to 3 minutes per side. Season with more salt, cayenne, and black pepper to taste, if desired. Transfer each fillet to a plate. Top each with half of the salsa. Serve immediately.

MANGO CUCUMBER SALSA

$1^1/2$ tablespoons fresh lime juice
$1^1/2$ teaspoons honey
1 cup $1/4$-inch mango cubes
$3/4$ cup $1/4$-inch unpeeled hothouse (English) cucumber cubes
$1/3$ cup minced red onion
$1^1/2$ teaspoons minced and seeded green jalapeño pepper
Salt

Whisk the lime juice and honey in a medium resealable container until well combined. Add the mango, cucumber, onion, and jalapeño and stir until well combined. Seal the container and refrigerate for at least 1 hour to let the flavors meld. Season with salt to taste. Serve cold or allow to come to room temperature.

Makes about $1^1/2$ cups; 6 servings
Each $1/4$-cup serving has: 30 calories, <1 g protein, 8 g carbohydrates, trace fat, trace saturated fat, 0 g cholesterol, <1 g fiber, 13 mg sodium

---

MAKES 2 SERVINGS

2 Each 2-Decadent-Disk serving (1 fillet with $1/4$ cup plus 1 tablespoon salsa) has: 201 calories, 23 g protein, 10 g carbohydrates, 7 g fat, 1 g saturated fat, 62 mg cholesterol, 1 g fiber, 212 mg sodium

PESTO PARMESAN-CRUSTED SALMON

2

Have you ever made pesto? It's astounding how much olive oil will soak into the herbs. Couple that with the fact that most pesto has pine nuts in it, and you have a sauce that is high in fat.

I used to eat pesto all of the time until I realized that. After years of missing it, I started creating what I called "almost-pesto" that I could use as part of a dish to eliminate the excess oil. This "almost-pesto" dish quickly became one of my favorites.

It's very important that the basil leaves are dry before you add them to the food processor. This way you'll ensure the perfect crispy topping.

Olive oil spray
Four 3^{1}/$_{2}$-ounce skinless salmon fillets, bones removed
Salt and pepper
1 slice whole-wheat bread
14 medium fresh basil leaves
1 medium garlic clove
1 tablespoon grated reduced-fat Parmesan

Preheat the oven to 400°F.

Lightly mist a small nonstick baking sheet with spray.

Season both sides of the salmon fillets with salt and pepper to taste.

Tear the bread into large pieces and put it in the bowl of a food processor fitted with a chopping blade. Add the basil, garlic, and Parmesan. Process until minced, about 1 minute. Transfer to a sheet of wax paper. Place one fillet on the crumbs, so the side that had the skin is face up. Press it into the crumbs to coat the bottom only. Flip it and place it on the prepared baking sheet, crumb side up. Repeat with the remaining 3 fillets, coating them and then placing them side by side, not touching, on the sheet. If crumbs remain, spoon them among the fillets, and then press them on. Bake, uncovered, for 10 to 12 minutes, or until the fillets are pale pink throughout. Serve immediately.

Can be made in 30 minutes or less / No more than 20 minutes hands-on prep time

MAKES 4 SERVINGS

2 Each 2-Decadent-Disk serving (1 fillet) has: 209 calories, 21 g protein, 5 g carbohydrates, 11 g fat, 2 g saturated fat, 60 mg cholesterol, <1 g fiber, 127 mg sodium

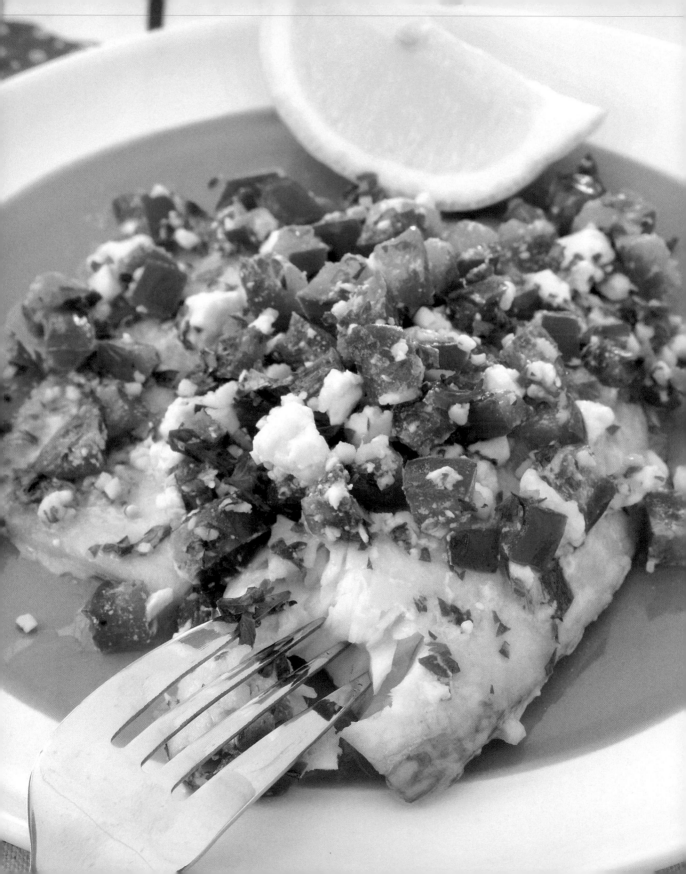

GREEK ROASTED TILAPIA FILLETS

Though I'm a fan of fish, I hadn't eaten much tilapia until working with *The Biggest Loser* contestants on their recipes. Many of them had given me recipes for tilapia. After going to the grocery store, I understood why. Not only is it a lot less expensive than most other fish (at least in my grocery stores), it has a really great, extremely subtle flavor and it doesn't dry out as easily as many other varieties of fish.

It reminds me a little bit of flounder, which is very prevalent on the East Coast, but virtually impossible to find on the West Coast. But tilapia is often also found frozen, sometimes even individually vacuum-packed, which is great because you can store it in your freezer and pull it out the day before you need it.

Here I've used tilapia to make one of my favorite fish preparations. And the best news? It's a cinch and you'll get a large portion for few calories. Just be sure to season the fillets directly with salt. That will really make a difference.

Olive oil spray
1 1/2 tablespoons minced fresh garlic
1 teaspoon extra virgin olive oil
1/3 cup chopped fresh flat-leaf parsley
2/3 cup seeded and chopped Roma tomatoes (see page 21)
1 3/4 ounces (about 1/3 cup) reduced-fat feta cheese, crumbled
1/2 pound tilapia fillets, bones removed
Salt and pepper

Preheat the oven to 400°F.

Lightly mist a medium ovenproof baking dish with spray.

Mix the garlic, olive oil, parsley, tomatoes, and feta in a medium bowl.

Lightly mist both sides of the tilapia fillets with spray, and then season both sides with salt and pepper to taste. Lay the fillets side by side, barely touching, in the prepared baking dish. Top evenly with the tomato mixture. Bake for 13 to 17 minutes, or until the tilapia flakes and is no longer translucent. Serve immediately.

Can be made in 30 minutes or less / No more than 20 minutes hands-on prep time

MAKES 2 SERVINGS

 Each 2-Decadent-Disk serving (1/2 recipe) has: 199 calories, 29 g protein, 6 g carbohydrates, 7 g fat, 3 g saturated fat, 65 mg cholesterol, 1 g fiber, 392 mg sodium

FRIED JUMBO SHRIMP

1 **2**

While I was growing up, we often went to a chain seafood restaurant near my parents' house. They had a kids' menu for kids under twelve. My mom always ordered for us off the kids' menu and then got fried jumbo shrimp for herself and shared some with us. She never ate much (I wish she had taught me that trick).

I remember, though, that a few months before my twelfth birthday, they started having an "all-you-can-eat fried shrimp special." I can't ever remember wanting my birthday to come so fast. All I could eat? Wow, that's a lot of shrimp. Let's just say that by the time I turned thirteen, I'd eaten way too much shrimp, and it showed. I still love it—in moderation, of course, and prepared just like this.

Note that the shrimp can be breaded up to one day in advance and stored in the refrig-

erator until you are ready to bake them. Also, if you've watched me on TV or cooked from my other books, you may notice that I often use whole-wheat panko bread crumbs. More often than not, I do use the whole-wheat ones these days. But in this recipe, I much prefer the plain white ones.

8 large (16–20 count) shrimp (about $^1/_2$ pound)
Olive oil spray
1 tablespoon unbleached all-purpose flour
1 teaspoon Creole seasoning
1 large egg white
1 teaspoon fat-free milk
$^1/_2$ cup panko bread crumbs
2 tablespoons jarred seafood cocktail sauce

Can be made in 30 minutes or less / No more than 20 minutes hands-on prep time

MAKES 8 SHRIMP; 2 SERVINGS OR 4 PORTIONS

1 Each 1-Decadent-Disk portion (2 shrimp plus 1$^1/_2$ teaspoons cocktail sauce) has: 96 calories, 13 g protein, 7 g carbohydrates, 1 g fat, trace saturated fat, 86 mg cholesterol, trace fiber, 240 mg sodium

2 Each 2-Decadent-Disk serving (4 shrimp plus 1 tablespoon cocktail sauce) has: 193 calories, 26 g protein, 15 g carbohydrates, 3 g fat, trace saturated fat, 172 mg cholesterol, trace fiber, 481 mg sodium

Peel the shrimp, but don't remove the tails. Butterfly the shrimp by cutting them down the back so they flatten but are not cut through. Rinse to clean them. Shake off any excess water, and then pat them dry with a paper towel.

Preheat the oven to 450°F.

Lightly mist a medium nonstick baking sheet with spray.

Mix the flour and Creole seasoning in a medium shallow bowl.

Pour the egg white into a second shallow bowl and add the milk. Lightly beat with a fork until well combined and slightly bubbly. Set the bowl next to the flour mixture.

Pour the bread crumbs into a third medium shallow bowl. Set the bowl next to the bowl with the egg.

Dip one shrimp into the flour mixture, coating it evenly on all sides. Shake off any excess flour. Next dip it into the egg mixture, followed by the bread crumbs. Shake off any excess bread crumbs and transfer the shrimp to the prepared baking sheet. Continue breading each shrimp, placing them side by side, not touching, on the baking sheet.

Bake for 5 minutes on one side, and then carefully flip them, being sure to leave the breading intact, and bake for another 4 to 6 minutes, or until the breading is crisp and the shrimp are plump and cooked through. Serve immediately with seafood cocktail sauce.

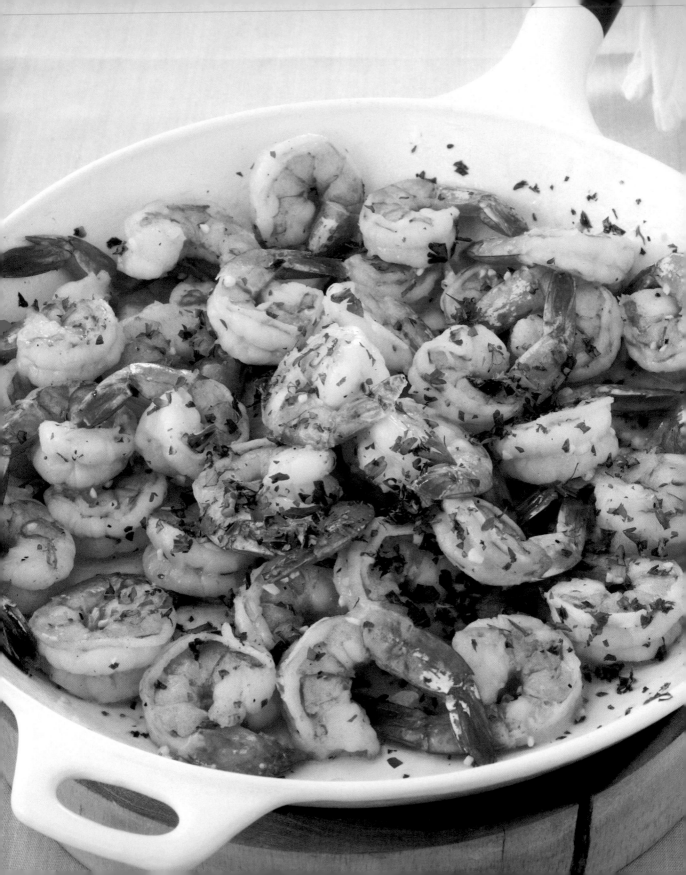

SKINNY SCAMPI

2

Shrimp may be the perfect "diet food." Even if it were fattening, I'd consider eating it. Couple it with fresh garlic, my favorite seasoning, and how can you go wrong?

Whatever you do, when you start preparing this recipe, make sure you have all of your ingredients measured and ready to go before adding the wine and lemon juice to the pan. Though it's always recommended that you prep everything in advance, it's not always key. Here, it definitely is or the wine and lemon juice will evaporate while you're off measuring—not only could it be detrimental to the taste, but you could easily burn your pan.

Also, notice that the shrimp are cooked in batches. It's important not to cut corners on that. Overcrowding the pan will not yield the same better-than-at-your-local-restaurant results.

1¼ pounds medium (31–40 count) shrimp, peeled (tails left on) and deveined
1 teaspoon extra virgin olive oil
¼ teaspoon salt, or to taste
Black pepper
6 garlic cloves, minced (about 2½ tablespoons)

¼ cup dry white wine
2 tablespoons fresh lemon juice
2 tablespoons light butter (stick, not tub)
2 tablespoons minced fresh parsley

Toss the shrimp with the olive oil, salt, and pepper to taste in a medium bowl.

Place a large nonstick skillet over high heat. When the skillet is hot, put in half of the shrimp. Cook, stirring occasionally, until they are just pink on both sides, 2 to 3 minutes. Add half of the garlic and cook, stirring constantly, until the shrimp are lightly browned on the outside and cooked through, 1 to 2 minutes. Transfer the shrimp to a platter and cover to keep hot. Repeat with the remaining shrimp and garlic. Add them to the platter and cover.

Add the wine and lemon juice to the pan. When the liquid is reduced by half, 1 to 2 minutes, turn the heat to low and add the butter and 1 tablespoon parsley. Use a wooden spoon to stir until the butter is melted completely, 30 seconds to 1 minute. Spoon the sauce over the shrimp and toss well, then garnish with the remaining parsley. Serve immediately.

Can be made in 30 minutes or less / No more than 20 minutes hands-on prep time

MAKES 4 SERVINGS

2 Each 2-Decadent-Disk serving (¼ recipe) has: 207 calories, 29 g protein, 4 g carbohydrates, 7 g fat, 2 g saturated fat, 223 mg cholesterol, trace fiber, 405 mg sodium

You save: 514 calories, 52 g fat, 22 g saturated fat

Traditional serving: 721 calories, 32 g protein, 6 g carbohydrates, 59 g fat, 24 g saturated fat, 311 mg cholesterol, trace fiber, 650 mg sodium

starchy sides

ONE POTATO, TWO POTATO, STUFFING and more: an entire chapter brimming with potato dishes that won't set you back. Meat-and-potatoes lovers, this one's for you!

Carbs have gotten a bad rap for a long time, but they are coming back into favor for their many benefits. As long as you're filling up on whole grains and natural ingredients, such as good old-fashioned potatoes, you will be fueling your workouts and giving yourself an energy boost. So whether you've been dying for otherwise off-limits fries or have a small craving for stuffing, this chapter will put you on the right track to eating those foods in a smart way. After all, mashed potatoes are as comforting as any food can be. Why even try to live without them? I certainly don't.

1 Pineapple Fried Rice

1 **2** Good-Enough-for-Thanksgiving Sausage-Cranberry Stuffing

1 Green Chile and Cheddar Croquettes

1 Parmesan-Garlic Mashed Potato Pancakes

1 **2** Crinkle-Cut Fries

1 **2** Italian Seasoned Fries

1 **2** Horseradish Smashed Potatoes

1 **2** Oven-Roasted Potatoes, Peppers, and Sweet Onions

1 **2** Chipotle Mashed Sweet Potatoes

1 **2** Tart Cherry Couscous

1 **2** Taboulied Couscous

PINEAPPLE FRIED RICE

We constantly hear that Chinese food is bad for us. It is often made with "bad oils" and lots of them, even when it's not deep-fried. Plus it tends to have an astronomical amount of sodium. I used to be so bummed because I really love it. But now that I can re-create dishes like Chinese Pepper Steak (page 115), Sweet-and-Sour Chicken Bowl (page 147), Spicy Szechuan Steak (page 114), and various fried rice dishes, I don't even miss it.

Though this particular fried rice dish might be more commonly found on a menu at a Thai restaurant, I always associate fried rice with Chinese food. And I often serve this fried rice with my Chinese favorites. Not only does it add a bit of variety, but the tomatoes and pineapple allow me to have a bigger serving than other rice dishes without a huge addition of fat or calories.

$1/2$ teaspoon extra virgin olive oil
2 teaspoons minced peeled fresh ginger
2 teaspoons minced fresh garlic
1 cup cooked and cooled long-grain white rice
$1/4$ cup finely chopped whole green onion
$1/2$ cup diced fresh pineapple
$1/2$ cup seeded and diced tomato (see page 21)
$1 1/2$ teaspoons lower-sodium soy sauce
1 teaspoon curry powder

Place a medium nonstick wok or skillet over medium-high heat. Put in the olive oil, ginger, and garlic. Cook, stirring constantly, until the garlic begins to soften, 1 to 2 minutes.

Next, stir in the rice, green onion, pineapple, tomato, soy sauce, and curry powder. Continue cooking, stirring occasionally, until all of the ingredients are heated through, 1 to 2 minutes. Serve immediately.

Can be made in 30 minutes or less / No more than 20 minutes hands-on prep time

MAKES 2 CUPS; 3 SERVINGS

Each 1-Decadent-Disk serving ($2/3$ cup) has: 104 calories, 2 g protein, 21 g carbohydrates, 1 g fat, <1 g saturated fat, 0 mg cholesterol, 2 g fiber, 95 mg sodium

GOOD-ENOUGH-FOR-THANKSGIVING SAUSAGE-CRANBERRY STUFFING

1 **2**

Around Thanksgiving time, I tend to get inundated with fan letters asking if I have a recipe for low-carb stuffing. My response is always the same: my idea of low-carb stuffing is eating plenty of turkey, plenty of salad, coleslaw (see Colorful Coleslaw, page 189), or other healthy, low-carb sides, then eating just a little bit of stuffing made with real bread. Here, I lower the carbs even further by adding plenty of homemade sausage, and I help fill you up by using wheat bread instead of white. Just be sure to pick a fluffy wheat bread, not a grainy one.

Though this stuffing is amazing made according to the recipe, I do actually put it in the turkey on Thanksgiving. When it's baked in the turkey, I truly believe that it is better than any stuffing I've ever had. In fact, I'm so convinced, I served it to one of the producers of *Seinfeld* and his family when he hired me to cook his Thanksgiving dinner for the first time in my early days of catering. He tipped me more than I'd ever been tipped before and his family kept raving.

Note that I recommend lower-sodium (or reduced-sodium) chicken broth, not low-sodium. Made with truly low-sodium broth, this dish is not worth making.

This stuffing can be made up to one day in advance. If you're putting it in a turkey, do not stuff the turkey until just before you are ready to cook it.

Butter-flavored cooking spray
12 slices whole-wheat bread (about 70 calories per slice)
Olive oil spray
1 recipe Sweet and Slim Italian Sausage (page 130), uncooked and unshaped
1 1/2 cups finely chopped sweet onion
1 cup finely chopped celery
1 tablespoon minced fresh garlic
1/2 cup dried cranberries
1 tablespoon finely chopped fresh sage
1 1/4 to 1 1/2 cups fat-free lower-sodium (not low-sodium) chicken broth, divided
2 tablespoons light butter, melted

MAKES ABOUT 7 CUPS; 10 SERVINGS OR 20 PORTIONS

1 Each 1-Decadent-Disk portion (slightly heaping 1/3 cup) has: 102 calories, 8 g protein, 14 g carbohydrates, 2 g fat, <1 g saturated fat, 16 mg cholesterol, 2 g fiber, 269 mg sodium

2 Each 2-Decadent-Disk serving (heaping 2/3 cup) has: 205 calories, 15 g protein, 29 g carbohydrates, 4 g fat, 1 g saturated fat, 32 mg cholesterol, 4 g fiber, 538 mg sodium

You save: 309 calories, 34 g fat, 7 g saturated fat

Traditional serving: 514 calories, 16 g protein, 27 g carbohydrates, 38 g fat, 8 g saturated fat, 56 mg cholesterol, 2 g fiber, 924 mg sodium

Preheat the oven to 300°F.

Lightly mist a 2½ to 3-quart ovenproof ceramic or glass casserole dish with butter-flavored cooking spray.

Place the slices of bread side by side in a single layer (they should not overlap) on a large nonstick baking sheet. Toast in the oven for 14 to 16 minutes per side, until the slices are dry (not at all soft in the center), but not more than very lightly browned.

Meanwhile, place a large nonstick skillet over medium-high heat. When the skillet is hot, lightly mist it with olive oil spray and put in the sausage mixture. Cook, breaking the sausage into bite-sized chunks, until no longer pink, 3 to 5 minutes. Transfer the sausage to a large mixing bowl.

Turn the heat to medium, respray the pan, and put in the onions. Cook for 5 minutes, and then add the celery and garlic. Continue cooking until the celery is bright green and starts to soften slightly, 7 to 10 minutes. Add the celery mixture to the sausage.

Increase the oven temperature to 350°F.

When the bread is cooled enough to touch, cut each slice into 9 squares.

Add the bread, cranberries, and sage to the sausage mixture and stir until well combined. Drizzle 1 cup broth slowly over the top and stir it in until the liquid is absorbed. Slowly drizzle the butter over the top and stir that in.

Transfer the stuffing to the prepared casserole dish. Drizzle the remaining ¼ cup broth for a drier stuffing or ½ cup for a moister stuffing over the top. Cover and bake for 30 minutes. Remove the cover and bake for another 10 to 15 minutes, until the bread is golden brown and the stuffing is hot throughout. Remove from the oven and let stand for 10 minutes.

GREEN CHILE AND CHEDDAR CROQUETTES

When I was working on recipes for my TV show, *Healthy Decadence,* we were attempting to make bacon and Cheddar mashed potatoes. They kept turning a grayish purple. It was the strangest thing. We'd cook the bacon, add the onions, and then mix them into the mashed potatoes along with the cheese, and time after time they turned this odd hue. The flavor was dead-on, but the color was weird and the potatoes were gummy. Obviously that wasn't going to fly.

We kept playing around and finally decided to make a bacon and Cheddar mashed potato gratin using the exact same ingredients. It was delicious. Then, I figured out that the potatoes got gummy and strangely colored only when we added the ingredients to the hot potatoes. If the potatoes were cooled, there was no problem. So you can learn from my mistake. When making these croquettes, be sure that the potatoes are no warmer than room temperature before adding the cheese.

For convenience, note that these potatoes (and most breaded foods) can be breaded a day in advance of baking and serving. Store them in an airtight container in a single layer in the refrigerator.

1½ pounds baking potatoes (about 3 medium potatoes), peeled and cut into 1-inch pieces
2 tablespoons fat-free half-and-half
1 tablespoon light butter, softened
2½ ounces (about 1¼ cups) finely shredded Cabot's 75% Light Cheddar cheese, or your favorite low-fat Cheddar
¼ cup chopped canned green chiles
1 teaspoon garlic powder, divided
Salt
Black pepper
Olive oil spray (real olive oil, not Pam)
1 large egg white
1½ teaspoons fat-free milk
⅓ cup plain dried bread crumbs

Cook the potatoes in a pot of boiling salted water until tender, 12 to 15 minutes. Drain.

Transfer the potatoes to a medium mixing bowl and mash with a potato masher until no lumps remain. Cool to room temperature, about 30 minutes.

Add the half-and-half, butter, cheese, chiles, and ½ teaspoon garlic powder. Stir until well combined, and then season with salt and pepper to taste. Cover with plastic wrap and refrigerate for about 1 hour, or until cooled.

MAKES ABOUT 24 CROQUETTES; 8 SERVINGS

Each 1-Decadent-Disk serving (3 croquettes) has: 102 calories, 5 g protein, 16 g carbohydrates, 2 g fat, <1 g saturated fat, 5 mg cholesterol, 1 g fiber, 276 mg sodium

You save: 73 calories, 9 g fat, 2 g saturated fat

Traditional serving: 175 calories, 5 g protein, 14 g carbohydrates, 11 g fat, 3 g saturated fat, 39 mg cholesterol, 1 g fiber, 319 mg sodium

Preheat the oven to 450°F.

Lightly mist a medium nonstick baking sheet with spray.

Place a large sheet of wax paper or parchment paper on a flat work surface. Use a 1½-inch cookie scoop or two large spoons to divide the mixture into 24 portions (about 2 tablespoons each). Roll each portion with your hands to form a perfect ball, and then return it to the paper.

Put the egg white and milk in a small deep bowl. Use a fork to beat it until well combined.

Put the bread crumbs, the remaining garlic powder, and ⅛ teaspoon salt in a medium resealable plastic bag. Seal the bag and shake to mix.

Dip the balls one by one into the egg mixture to coat, letting any excess drip off, and then coat them in the bread crumb mixture. Place side by side, not touching, on the prepared baking sheet. Lightly mist the tops with spray. Bake for 5 minutes, then carefully flip them. Bake for another 4 to 6 minutes, or until lightly browned on the outside and heated through; if the cheese starts melting and deforming them, remove from the oven. Lightly mist them with spray and serve immediately.

PARMESAN-GARLIC MASHED POTATO PANCAKES

Though I was convinced that by age fifteen I had been on every diet on the planet, I was never even tempted to jump on the "low-carb" bandwagon. There was just something about a diet that said you could have fat-laden, chemical-laden, "low-carb" tortilla chips, but you couldn't have an apple, that never made sense to me. Well, that and the fact that I'd long since committed to living *The Most Decadent Diet Ever!* by the time the low-carb "thing" was trendy. But recipes like these, which I've been enjoying for years, make it clear why I never would have been able to stick to a low-carb diet long-term. I love potatoes. And I love "fried" foods. These pancakes combine the two flavors and are a great accompaniment to lots of meat dishes. And when two pancakes have only 100 calories, how can you go wrong?

1¹/₂ pounds baking potatoes (about 3 medium potatoes), peeled and cut into 1-inch pieces
¹/₂ cup fat-free half-and-half
2 tablespoons light butter, melted
2 tablespoons grated reduced-fat Parmesan
1 tablespoon finely chopped fresh parsley
1 teaspoon minced fresh garlic
Salt and pepper
Olive oil spray (real olive oil, not Pam)

Cook the potatoes in a pot of boiling salted water until tender, 12 to 15 minutes. Drain.

Transfer the potatoes to a medium mixing bowl. Mash slightly with a fork. Add the half-and-half, butter, Parmesan, parsley, and garlic. Use an electric mixer fitted with beaters to beat until fluffy. Season with salt and pepper to taste. Cool to room temperature.

Preheat the oven to 450°F.

Line a large baking sheet with parchment paper. Lightly mist it with spray.

Place a sheet of wax paper or parchment paper on a flat work surface. Divide the potato mixture into 14 portions, form each into a 2-inch ball (use a 2-inch cookie scoop, if you have one), and place them on the paper. Transfer the balls to the prepared baking sheet, working in batches, if necessary, spaced far enough apart (about 4 inches) to double in diameter without touching (the pancakes will spread slightly). Then use the back of a large spoon to flatten each ball into a 3-inch circle.

Lightly mist the tops with spray and sprinkle lightly with salt. Cook for 8 minutes, then carefully flip them. Lightly mist the tops with spray and sprinkle lightly with salt, or to taste. Cook until lightly browned on the outside and heated through, another 4 to 6 minutes. Serve immediately.

No more than 20 minutes hands-on prep time

MAKES 14 PANCAKES; 7 SERVINGS

 Each 1-Decadent-Disk serving (2 pancakes) has: 99 calories, 3 g protein, 18 g carbohydrates, 2 g fat, 1 g saturated fat, 6 mg cholesterol, 1 g fiber, 179 mg sodium

CRINKLE-CUT FRIES

1 **2**

My high school served crinkle-cut fries and pizza every single day, along with a more sensible option. Needless to say, the French fries and pizza won. I remember being so resentful that I was fat, yet so many kids would eat plate after plate of fries followed by cupcakes for dessert.

For years, I completely gave up the fries. But thanks to this version, they're back in my diet. And I can enjoy a food that plenty of others do, guilt free.

A fan recently wrote to me on MySpace and told me that she loved the French fries I make. She said that she made them with extra light olive oil instead of extra virgin and wanted to know how many calories and how much fat the substitution would save her. Do you know the answer to that? If not, the answer is zero. In the case of extra light olive oil, the "light" refers to the flavor, not the fat or calories. Using an extra light oil only takes away that great, strong taste that extra virgin olive oil packs. She tried the fries again with the extra virgin and said she loved them even more.

Please note: you'll need a crinkle-cutting tool for this recipe. The good news is that they tend to cost only a few dollars (see page 19).

Olive oil spray
2 pounds baking potatoes
$^1/_4$ teaspoon salt, plus more to taste, if desired
$1^1/_2$ teaspoons extra virgin olive oil

Preheat the oven to 400°F.

Lightly mist a medium nonstick baking sheet with spray.

Use a crinkle cutter to peel the potatoes by cutting close to the edges on each side and each end. Discard the peels. Then use the crinkle cutter to cut the peeled potatoes into $^1/_3$-inch-thick sticks. (They will vary in length.) After discarding the peels and any deformed cuts, you should have approximately 1 pound (about 4 cups) remaining.

Toss the potato sticks with $^1/_4$ teaspoon salt and the olive oil. Then place them in a single layer, not touching, on the prepared baking sheet. Bake for 15 minutes, and then flip them and bake for another 16 to 18 minutes, or until they are just crisp on the outside and tender on the inside. Season with additional salt to taste, if desired, and serve immediately.

No more than 20 minutes hands-on prep time

MAKES 2 SERVINGS OR 4 PORTIONS

1 Each 1-Decadent-Disk portion ($^1/_4$ recipe) has: 105 calories, 2 g protein, 20 g carbohydrates, 2 g fat, trace saturated fat, 0 mg cholesterol, 2 g fiber, 152 mg sodium

2 Each 2-Decadent-Disk serving ($^1/_2$ recipe) has: 210 calories, 5 g protein, 41 g carbohydrates, 4 g fat, <1 g saturated fat, 0 mg cholesterol, 3 g fiber, 304 mg sodium

You save: 201 calories, 24 g fat, 5 g saturated fat

Traditional serving: 412 calories, 4 g protein, 35 g carbohydrates, 28 g fat, 6 g saturated fat, 0 mg cholesterol, 3 g fiber, 775 mg sodium

ITALIAN SEASONED FRIES

🟊 1 🟊 2

One of the great things about making your own fries (in addition to their being much less fattening than those you eat out) is that you can tailor them to your preferences using herbs and seasonings. Feeling like some garlic fries today? Simply sprinkle them with some garlic, salt (or garlic salt), and a touch of parsley. Add some Parmesan and crushed red pepper flakes and you have these Italian fries. Like spicy Cajun fries? Hit them up with some Cajun seasoning. Or sprinkle them with some fresh garlic and rosemary and you'll be in for a different treat. The important thing to remember is that you need only a touch of olive oil to create the perfect fries.

You can bake these fries directly on a good nonstick pan if you don't have parchment paper. The parchment simply ensures that the ingredients won't stick in case your pan has lost its nonstick property over time.

1 medium (8$\frac{1}{2}$-to 9-ounce) baking potato, peeled and cut into sticks about $\frac{1}{2}$ inch thick
$\frac{1}{2}$ teaspoon extra virgin olive oil
1$\frac{1}{2}$ teaspoons grated reduced-fat Parmesan
$\frac{1}{2}$ teaspoon finely chopped fresh flat-leaf parsley
$\frac{1}{8}$ teaspoon garlic powder
$\frac{1}{8}$ teaspoon crushed red pepper flakes
Salt

Preheat the oven to 450°F.

Line a medium nonstick baking sheet with parchment paper.

Toss the potato sticks with the olive oil, Parmesan, parsley, garlic, red pepper flakes, and salt to taste. Place them in a single layer, not touching, on the prepared baking sheet. Bake for 8 minutes, flip them, and bake for another 10 to 12 minutes, or until the potatoes are tender on the inside and have some browned spots on them, but are not completely browned. Serve immediately.

Can be made in 30 minutes or less / No more than 20 minutes hands-on prep time

MAKES 1 SERVING OR 2 PORTIONS

🟊 1 Each 1-Decadent-Disk portion ($\frac{1}{2}$ recipe) has: 97 calories, 2 g protein, 19 g carbohydrates, 2 g fat, trace saturated fat, 2 mg cholesterol, 2 g fiber, 34 mg sodium

🟊 2 Each 2-Decadent-Disk serving (1 recipe) has: 195 calories, 5 g protein, 38 g carbohydrates, 3 g fat, trace saturated fat, 4 mg cholesterol, 3 g fiber, 69 mg sodium

HORSERADISH SMASHED POTATOES
1 **2**

Growing up, I never liked mashed potatoes. Not even a tiny bit. Looking back, it's so bizarre, because I could truly eat them at every meal now.

The turning point came when an ex-boyfriend and I went to this cute little restaurant that had an organic garden in the backyard. They grew all of their own herbs and many of their veggies. I can't even remember what I ordered but whatever it was came with a side of basil mashed potatoes that I will never forget. I don't even know why I tried them perhaps because I love basil so much—but that's when my love affair with mashed potatoes began. Since that time, I've probably created at least twenty or more varieties. This is one of the simpler ones, and it is excellent with many dishes. You may want to try it with Salisbury Steaks with Rich Brown Gravy (page 116) or Mini-Meatloaves (page 128).

Please note that the 1-Decadent-Disk portion here is on the small side. But if you're like me, sometimes a little bit is plenty. I tend to eat only a 1-Decadent-Disk portion ever. I usually fill up on protein and salad and then just dive into a few bites (^{1}/3 of a cup isn't so small). That leaves me room for dessert. If you're not a dessert person, then a 2-Decadent-Disk serving of smashed potatoes just might be perfect.

1 pound unpeeled red potatoes (about 4 large red potatoes), cut into 1-inch pieces
1 teaspoon salt, plus more to taste
3 tablespoons fat-free half-and-half
2^1/2 tablespoons light butter
1 tablespoon bottled horseradish, or more to taste
Black pepper

Place the potatoes in a medium pot. Add enough cold water to cover the potatoes by 2 inches. Place the pot over high heat and add 1 teaspoon salt. Bring the water to a boil and cook the potatoes, covered, until tender, 20 to 25 minutes.

Just before the potatoes are cooked, combine the half-and-half, butter, and horseradish in a medium microwave-safe bowl. Microwave on low for 1 to 2 minutes, until the butter is melted.

Drain the potatoes and transfer to a medium mixing bowl. Use a potato masher or large fork to smash them slightly. Pour in the half-and-half mixture and continue to mix until the potatoes are smashed, leaving some lumps. Season with salt and pepper to taste. Serve immediately.

No more than 20 minutes hands-on prep time

MAKES ABOUT 2^1/4 CUPS; 5 PORTIONS
1 Each 1-Decadent-Disk portion (about ^{1}/3 cup) has: 97 calories, 2 g protein, 16 g carbohydrates, 3 g fat, 2 g saturated fat, 8 mg cholesterol, 2 g fiber, 125 mg sodium
2 Each 2-Decadent-Disk serving (heaping ^{2}/3 cup) has: 194 calories, 4 g protein, 32 g carbohydrates, 7 g fat, 4 g saturated fat, 16 mg cholesterol, 3 g fiber, 251 mg sodium
You save: 77 calories, 7 g fat, 4 g saturated fat
Traditional serving: 271 calories, 5 g protein, 34 g carbohydrates, 14 g fat, 8 g saturated fat, 35 mg cholesterol, 3 g fiber, 200 mg sodium

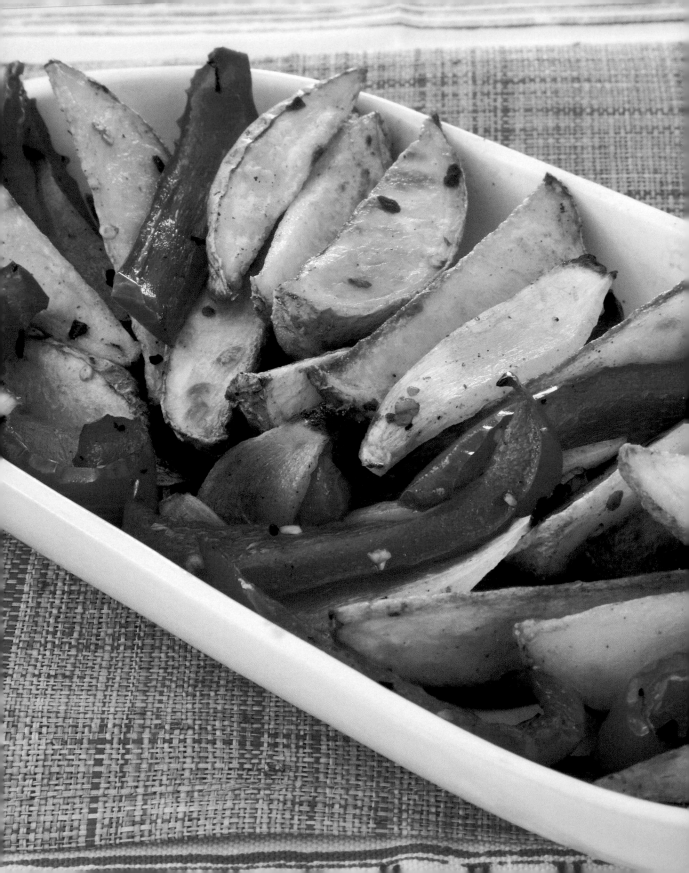

OVEN-ROASTED POTATOES, PEPPERS, AND SWEET ONIONS

1 **2**

Though this dish roasts for 30 minutes, I find it incredibly simple to make on those nights I just don't really feel like cooking. Since I can throw it together in less than 5 minutes, and it combines my starch with my veggies, it's one of my fallback side dishes. Well, that and I just love the flavors. It always tastes so fattening to me.

If you're not following *The Most Decadent Diet Ever!* to the letter, feel free to add more onions to this dish. I usually add 1/4 cup more, which has only 16 calories. Now that I've moved into a more mellow phase of the plan and don't actually count calories, I don't need to worry and sometimes I just crave a few more.

2 small (6-ounce) baking potatoes, each cut into
    8 wedges lengthwise
1 medium red or green bell pepper or a
    combination, cut into $3/4$-inch-wide strips (see
    page 20)
$3/4$ cup $3/4$-inch-wide sweet onion strips
$1 1/2$ teaspoons extra virgin olive oil
1 teaspoon minced fresh garlic
$1/4$ teaspoon paprika
$1/4$ teaspoon crushed red pepper flakes
$1/8$ teaspoon salt, plus more to taste
Black pepper

Preheat the oven to 400°F.

Combine the potatoes, bell pepper, onion, olive oil, garlic, paprika, red pepper flakes, and 1/8 teaspoon salt in a medium glass or plastic mixing bowl. Toss until the potatoes are evenly seasoned, then transfer in a single layer, not touching, to a large nonstick baking sheet. Bake for 15 minutes, and then flip and bake for another 12 to 15 minutes, until the potatoes are tender when pierced with a fork. Season with additional salt and pepper to taste, if desired. Serve immediately.

No more than 20 minutes hands-on prep time

MAKES 2 SERVINGS OR 4 PORTIONS

1 Each 1-Decadent-Disk portion (1/4 recipe) has: 100 calories, 19 g carbohydrates, 2 g protein, 2 g fat, <1 g saturated fat, 0 mg cholesterol, 3 g fiber, 79 mg sodium

2 Each 2-Decadent-Disk serving (1/2 recipe) has: 201 calories, 5 g protein, 39 g carbohydrates, 4 g fat, <1 g saturated fat, 0 mg cholesterol, 6 g fiber, 158 mg sodium

CHIPOTLE MASHED SWEET POTATOES

I'm sure you've heard by now that trainers and nutritionists recommend sweet potatoes over white potatoes because they have more nutrients and fiber. Although I agree, I definitely prefer white potatoes more often than not. This dish, however, is one where I truly enjoy the taste of sweet potatoes. The fiery chipotle peppers in adobo give them great depth—and they are a heck of a lot less fattening when prepared this way.

Look for the chipotle peppers in adobo in the international section of your grocery store. They're usually found with the Mexican foods such as green chiles.

2^1/$_2$ pounds red-skinned sweet potatoes (about 3 large potatoes), peeled and cut into 1-inch pieces
^{1}/$_4$ cup fat-free half-and-half
3 tablespoons light butter
1 to 2 tablespoons finely chopped canned chipotle peppers in adobo (see page 16)
Salt and pepper

Cook the potatoes in a pot of boiling salted water until tender, about 20 minutes.

Just before the potatoes are cooked, combine the half-and-half and butter in a small microwave-safe bowl. Microwave on low for about 1 minute, or until the butter melts.

Drain the potatoes and transfer them to a medium mixing bowl. Add the butter mixture and 1 tablespoon chipotle peppers. Beat with an electric mixer fitted with beaters until fluffy. Season with the remaining chipotle peppers, if desired, and season with salt and pepper to taste. Serve immediately.

No more than 20 minutes hands-on prep time

MAKES 4 CUPS; 5 SERVINGS OR 10 PORTIONS

Each 1-Decadent-Disk portion (scant ^{1}/$_2$ cup) has: 98 calories, 2 g protein, 19 g carbohydrates, 2 g fat, 1 g saturated fat, 5 mg cholesterol, 3 g fiber, 90 mg sodium

Each 2-Decadent-Disk serving (heaping ^{3}/$_4$ cup) has: 196 calories, 3 g protein, 39 g carbohydrates, 4 g fat, 2 g saturated fat, 9 mg cholesterol, 6 g fiber, 181 mg sodium

TART CHERRY COUSCOUS

1 **2**

One of the fun parts of my job is that I am often sent samples of new foods on the market along with lots of cooking equipment to test. Companies hope that I will include them in my magazine articles, books, or TV shows.

When the products are great, I do try to spread the word. The funny thing is that I'm often on the same list as magazine editors. When companies send something to magazines, they want to make sure to send enough to feed the entire office. I was recently shipped enough sample-sized protein bars from one company to fill six vases. When guests came, I offered them a handful on the way out the door.

Another item I recently received was a giant bag of dried tart cherries. They were so good. And I'd recently realized that they're chock-full of antioxidants, so I decided to start incorporating them in recipes. I made a black rice dish, a cherry balsamic chicken dish, and this couscous, which everyone loved. Though I've always loved tart cherries, I hadn't cooked with them much before and didn't realize just how versatile and scrumptious they are.

1 cup whole-wheat couscous
$\frac{1}{2}$ cup finely chopped pitted dried tart cherries
$\frac{1}{3}$ cup finely chopped whole green onions
$\frac{1}{4}$ cup fresh lime juice
$\frac{1}{4}$ cup chopped fresh flat-leaf parsley
1 tablespoon plus 1 teaspoon extra virgin olive oil
2 teaspoons to 1 tablespoon minced fresh garlic
Salt and pepper

Bring $1\frac{1}{2}$ cups water to a boil in a small saucepan. Stir in the couscous and cherries. Cover the pan, remove from the heat, and let stand, covered, for 5 minutes. Then fluff the couscous with a fork. Transfer the couscous to a medium mixing bowl and stir in the onions, lime juice, parsley, olive oil, and garlic. Season with salt and pepper to taste. Serve immediately.

Can be made in 30 minutes or less / No more than 20 minutes hands-on prep time

MAKES 4$\frac{1}{4}$ CUPS; 4 SERVINGS OR 8 PORTIONS

1 Each 1-Decadent-Disk portion (about $\frac{1}{2}$ cup) has: 103 calories, 2 g protein, 19 g carbohydrates, 2 g fat, trace saturated fat, 0 mg cholesterol, 4 g fiber, 3 mg sodium

2 Each 2-Decadent-Disk serving (about 1 cup) has: 206 calories, 5 g protein, 38 g carbohydrates, 5 g fat, <1 g saturated fat, 0 mg cholesterol, 8 g fiber, 6 mg sodium

TABOULIED COUSCOUS

1 **2**

I was recently watching a TV show where Shaquille O'Neal ("Shaq") was intervening at a Florida school to help a group of students get in shape. In one of the episodes, he had a chef changing the cafeteria menus to take away the junk food and add more nutritious options. The chef suggested a couscous dish and Shaq lightly poked fun at him, saying that white people eat couscous.

Trust me, no matter what your skin color, you should try this dish. Whole-wheat couscous is such a great grain, because it never really seems dry even when you don't add a lot of oil or dressing. Most pasta requires a lot, but couscous doesn't. In this dish, I've used plenty of flat-leaf parsley and the flavors of tabouli to create one of my favorite summer (or anytime!) side dishes.

1 cup dry whole-wheat couscous
¼ cup plus 1 tablespoon fresh lemon juice
¼ cup finely chopped fresh flat-leaf parsley
3 tablespoons finely chopped whole green onion
2 tablespoons finely chopped fresh mint
1 tablespoon plus 1 teaspoon extra virgin olive oil
Salt and pepper

Cook the couscous according to package directions, omitting any butter or oil.

Stir together the couscous, lemon juice, parsley, green onion, mint, and olive oil in a medium mixing bowl until well combined. Season with salt and pepper to taste. Serve immediately, or refrigerate in an airtight container for up to 3 days.

Can be made in 30 minutes or less / No more than 20 minutes hands-on prep time

MAKES 3 CUPS; 3 SERVINGS OR 6 PORTIONS

1 Each 1-Decadent-Disk portion (½ cup) has: 104 calories, 3 g protein, 17 g carbohydrates, 3 g fat, trace saturated fat, 0 mg cholesterol, 3 g fiber, 3 mg sodium

2 Each 2-Decadent-Disk serving (1 cup) has: 208 calories, 6 g protein, 33 g carbohydrates, 7 g fat, <1 g saturated fat, 0 mg cholesterol, 5 g fiber, 7 mg sodium

You save: 91 calories, 11 g fat, 2 g saturated fat

Traditional serving: 195 calories, 4 g protein, 17 g carbohydrates, 14 g fat, 2 g saturated fat, 0 mg cholesterol, 5 g fiber, 30 mg sodium

GIRL (OR GUY) CANNOT LIVE ON chocolate alone. Sad, but true. Though I created an individual chocolate cake with 6 grams of fiber, I still need my veggies, and so do you. I urge you to eat at least five servings of fruits and vegetables per day. And trust me, more is even better. The more you fill up on veggies, the fewer cravings you'll have and the healthier you'll be.

In this chapter, I've taken some of the most popular veggies we're accustomed to eating and have given them some decadent qualities. When pairing them as part of a meal, be sure you're not going overboard. I try never to make more than two of the three major components (protein, carbs, veggie) in my meal overly decadent. If I'm eating a dessert, I'm not likely to have goat cheese on my vegetable. If I'm eating a baked potato with some fresh salsa, then I'll have a drippier meat dish and a gooey veggie. If I'm having a piece of fish and some seasoned fries, I definitely wouldn't hesitate to throw in some creamy coleslaw. You might want to keep this kind of balancing act in mind.

When ordering vegetables out, always be careful. I've ordered steamed veggies and had them come steamed, and then tossed in olive oil or melted butter. When you ask for them steamed, confirm that the kitchen won't be adding any fats or oils after cooking them.

When you are eating at home, throw a few on the grill tossed in just a touch of olive oil and balsamic vinegar (a little fresh garlic never hurts either), or nosh on them raw to your heart's content.

- Zucchini Boats with Goat Cheese and Sun-Dried Tomatoes
- Curried Veggie Skewers
- Roasted Ruby Tomatoes
- Broccoli Limone
- Sautéed Mushrooms au Vin
- Basil Butternut Smash
- Grilled Corn on the Cob
- Fried Zucchini
- Cilantro Queso Stuffed Mushrooms
- Asparagus with Sherry Shallot Vinaigrette
- Oven-Roasted Broccoli with Parmesan
- Snap Pea Stir-Fry
- Colorful Coleslaw

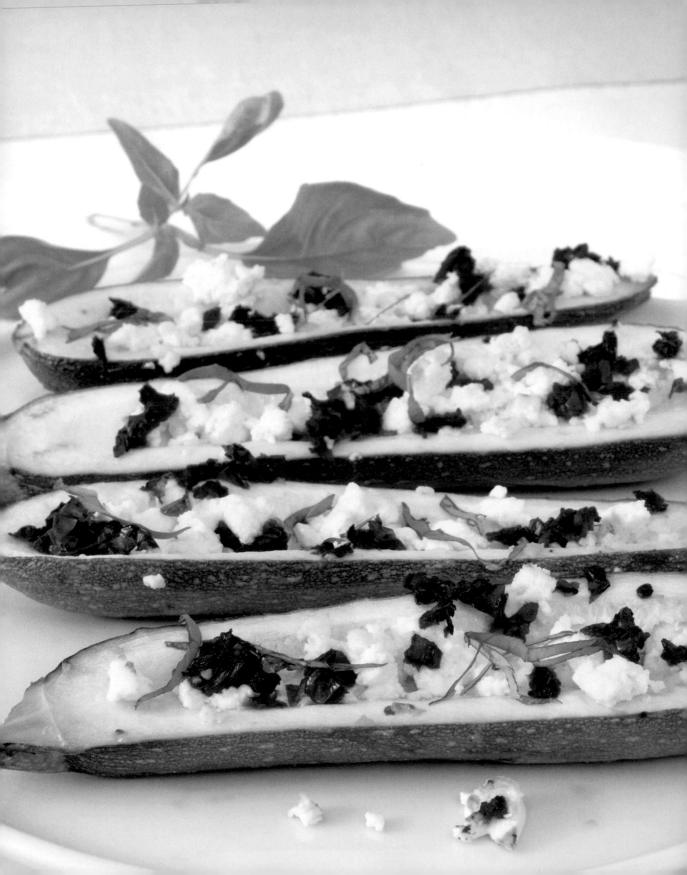

ZUCCHINI BOATS WITH GOAT CHEESE AND SUN-DRIED TOMATOES

①

I love to add sun-dried tomatoes to my salads or veggie dishes like this one for a flavor punch. Whatever you do, don't buy the ones that are packed in oil. Other varieties are sold either in airtight bags or in bulk. If they're soft when you buy them, simply add them to your dishes. If they're not soft, it's easy to soften them to prepare them for your recipe.

Just bring a small saucepan of water to a rolling boil. Stir in the tomatoes, and then turn off the heat. Let them sit in water, uncovered, for 5 minutes, or until tender. Drain them and they're ready to go.

If you can find it in your area, you can use light goat cheese in this recipe. Because it's not highly prevalent throughout the country, I wrote this recipe using the full-fat variety. Light goat cheese will save you another 33 calories and 3 grams of fat per serving.

Preheat the oven to 350°F.

Cut the zucchini in half lengthwise. Run the tip of a tablespoon down the center of each half, scraping out a shallow layer of the seeds. Lay the zucchini side by side, skin side down, on a small nonstick baking sheet and lightly mist each shell with spray. Sprinkle each zucchini half evenly with salt and pepper. Next, sprinkle the garlic evenly among them. Bake for 16 to 19 minutes, until tender. Sprinkle the goat cheese crumbles evenly over the zucchini, followed by the sun-dried tomatoes. Bake for another 4 to 6 minutes, or until the cheese is just barely starting to melt. Sprinkle the tops evenly with the basil, about $1/2$ teaspoon each. Serve immediately.

4 small zucchini

Olive oil spray

2 pinches of salt

2 pinches of black pepper

2 teaspoons minced fresh garlic

$3^1/_4$ ounces (scant $1/_2$ cup) crumbled goat cheese

2 tablespoons plus 2 teaspoons rehydrated chopped sun-dried tomatoes (not packed in oil)

1 tablespoon plus 1 teaspoon finely chopped fresh basil

No more than 20 minutes hands-on prep time

MAKES 8 BOATS; 4 SERVINGS

① Each 1-Decadent-Disk serving (2 boats) has: 102 calories, 7 g protein, 9 g carbohydrates, 5 g fat, 3 g saturated fat, 11 mg cholesterol, 3 g fiber, 188 mg sodium

You save: 80 calories, 9 g fat, 4 g saturated fat

Traditional serving: 182 calories, 8 g protein, 7 g carbohydrates, 14 g fat, 7 g saturated fat, 22 mg cholesterol, 2 g fiber, 257 mg sodium

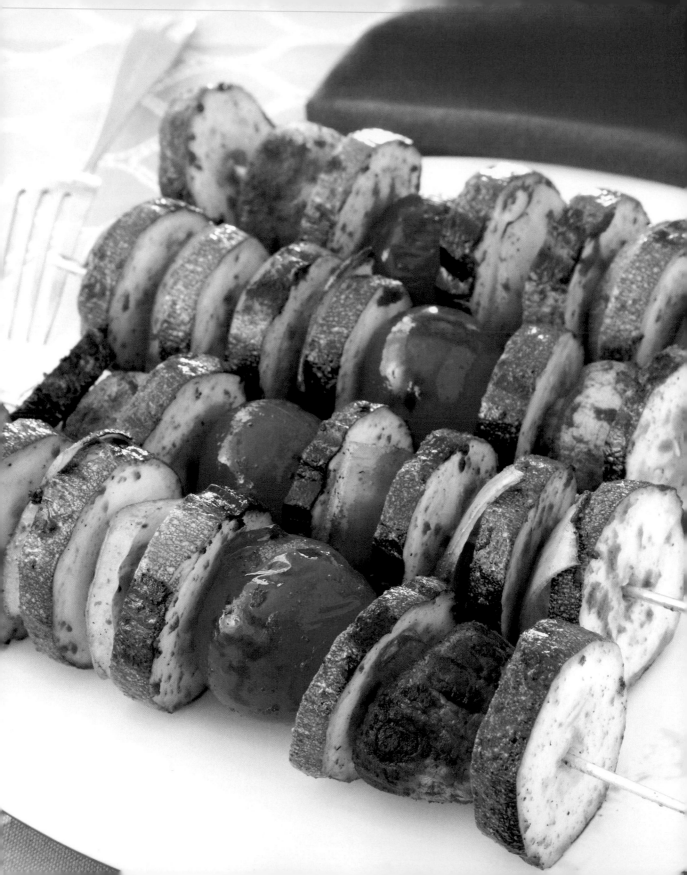

CURRIED VEGGIE SKEWERS

If you're really hungry, this recipe is a perfect answer. The portion is huge, and it takes only a few minutes to prepare. Granted, it may be too huge to eat in one sitting as an accompaniment to an entrée and side, but you can always eat half and have another ½-Decadent-Disk portion of something else. Or just eat them with an entrée. The large portion also accounts for why they contain 6 grams of fat.

If you love kebabs and skewered veggies as much as I do, it's worth purchasing metal skewers. You can get them at most cooking stores, in home improvement stores near the barbecue grills, and even at many grocery stores these days. Just be sure to get rustproof ones. If you prefer the wooden ones, they'll need to be soaked in water for at least ½ hour so they don't burn on the grill. The metal ones are good to go immediately.

Preheat a grill to high.

Combine the zucchini, onion, tomatoes, mushrooms, curry paste, and olive oil in a medium bowl. Toss until the veggies are well coated. Skewer 2 zucchini rounds, leaving a little space between the pieces so they will cook evenly. Next, skewer 2 onion squares, followed by 2 zucchini rounds, 1 tomato, 2 zucchini rounds, and 1 mushroom. On the same skewer, repeat. Then follow the same procedure to create a second skewer.

Turn the grill to low and place the skewers side by side on the grill. Grill for 5 to 6 minutes per side, or until some of the tomato skins begin to split and the other veggies are tender. Serve immediately.

24 zucchini rounds, ¼ inch thick
Eight 2-inch red onion squares
4 cherry tomatoes
4 small button mushrooms
1 teaspoon red curry paste
½ teaspoon extra virgin olive oil
2 metal skewers or 2 wooden skewers soaked in
    water for at least ½ hour

Can be made in 30 minutes or less / No more than 20 minutes hands-on prep time

MAKES 2 LARGE SKEWERS (OR 4 SMALL); 1 SERVING

Each 1-Decadent-Disk serving (2 large skewers) has: 104 calories, 4 g protein, 12 g carbohydrates, 6 g fat, <1 g saturated fat, 0 mg cholesterol, 4 g fiber, 185 mg sodium

You save: 87 calories, 10 g fat, 1 g saturated fat

Traditional serving: 190 calories, 3 g protein, 12 g carbohydrates, 16 g fat, 2 g saturated fat, 0 mg cholesterol, 3 g fiber, 300 mg sodium

ROASTED RUBY TOMATOES

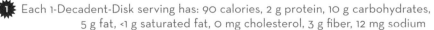

My dad loves tomatoes, and I definitely inherited that gene. I could eat a bowl or plate of tomatoes with a touch of sea salt any day. Here's a perked-up version of that summertime classic that feels even more substantial, especially in the winter months when we crave hot foods and tomatoes aren't at the peak of season. Plus, it doesn't hurt that they're a cinch to cook.

$^1/_2$ pound cherry tomatoes
1 teaspoon extra virgin olive oil
1$^1/_2$ teaspoons minced fresh garlic
Salt and pepper
1 tablespoon finely chopped fresh basil

Preheat the oven to 425°F.

Combine the tomatoes, olive oil, and garlic in a medium bowl. Toss until the tomatoes are evenly coated, and then season with salt and pepper to taste. Transfer in a single layer to a small nonstick baking sheet. Bake for 6 to 9 minutes, or until some of the tomato skins begin to split and the tomatoes are warmed through. Remove from the oven and sprinkle evenly with basil. Serve immediately.

Can be made in 30 minutes or less / No more than 20 minutes hands-on prep time

MAKES 1 SERVING

Each 1-Decadent-Disk serving has: 90 calories, 2 g protein, 10 g carbohydrates, 5 g fat, <1 g saturated fat, 0 mg cholesterol, 3 g fiber, 12 mg sodium

You save: 74 calories, 9 g fat, 1 g saturated fat

Traditional serving: 164 calories, 2 g protein, 10 g carbohydrates, 14 g fat, 2 g saturated fat, 0 mg cholesterol, 2 g fiber, 882 mg sodium

BROCCOLI LIMONE

I was recently asked to be the celebrity judge of a soyfoods cooking competition. I flew off to Iowa, where I'd never been, and attended the state fair. Boy, do they serve fried everything there, from cheese curds to fried Snickers!

Meanwhile, back at the culinary school where the competition was being held, one of the contestants, who owns a couple of health-food restaurants, had brought along his two adorable daughters. One was eight and the other was five. The eight-year-old was a black belt in karate, and the five-year-old was not far off. It was so cute to watch them do their forms (karate moves).

But the cutest part was when Steve, the dad, would say to the five-year-old, "What makes you fast?" She would excitedly respond, "Broccoli!" He'd say, "What makes you strong?" She'd jump in, "Lean protein like chicken!" Then he'd say, "What makes you smart?" She'd say, "Spinach!" The girls, as small as they were, really knew that healthy food was good, and that's what they ate through the entire weekend, except for a small treat at the fair. But healthy food was really what they wanted. Here's a recipe that, according to them, will help make you fast.

1 pound (about 6^1/$_2$ cups) broccoli florets
1 lemon, cut into 8 wedges

1 teaspoon fresh lemon juice
1 teaspoon extra virgin olive oil
1 teaspoon minced fresh garlic
^{1}/$_2$ teaspoon finely chopped fresh thyme
1 teaspoon light butter
Salt and pepper
1 teaspoon grated lemon zest

Place a steamer rack in a large pot. Fill the pot with water to just below the rack. Place the pot over high heat and bring the water to a boil. Put in the broccoli and lemon wedges, cover, and steam until the broccoli is crisp-tender, 5 to 7 minutes.

Meanwhile, put the lemon juice, olive oil, garlic, and thyme in a small nonstick skillet over medium heat. Cook, stirring often, until the garlic begins to soften, 2 to 3 minutes. Reduce the heat to low and add the butter. Stir until the butter is melted and immediately remove from the heat.

Discard the lemon wedges and transfer the broccoli to a large glass or plastic bowl. Pour the lemon mixture over the broccoli and toss until well combined. Season with salt and pepper to taste. Sprinkle the zest evenly over the top of the broccoli and serve immediately.

Can be made in 30 minutes or less / No more than 20 minutes hands-on prep time

MAKES 4 CUPS; 2 SERVINGS

Each 1-Decadent-Disk serving (2 cups) has: 96 calories, 7 g protein, 13 g carbohydrates, 4 g fat, 1 g saturated fat, 3 mg cholesterol, 7 g fiber, 77 mg sodium

You save: 110 calories, 14 g fat, 10 g saturated fat

Traditional serving: 206 calories, 5 g protein, 13 g carbohydrates, 18 g fat, 11 g saturated fat, 47 mg cholesterol, 7 g fiber, 365 mg sodium

SAUTÉED MUSHROOMS AU VIN

My assistant Stephanie loves mushrooms. Her dad should probably be credited with creating this recipe, though Stephanie wrote it with our healthy "most decadent" spin. She made it for a taste-testing party and my friends absolutely loved it. Though I owe Stephanie tons of thanks all of the time, I think this one deserves special mention.

2 teaspoons extra virgin olive oil
1¼ pounds sliced button mushrooms
⅓ cup finely chopped whole green onions
1 tablespoon minced fresh garlic
⅓ cup dry white wine
1 tablespoon Worcestershire sauce
Salt and pepper

Preheat a large skillet over medium-high heat. Put in the olive oil, mushrooms, green onions, and garlic. Cook, stirring occasionally, until the veggies become tender, 3 to 5 minutes. Add the wine and Worcestershire sauce. Cook until most of the liquid has evaporated, 6 to 9 minutes. Season with salt and pepper to taste. Serve immediately.

Can be made in 30 minutes or less / No more than 20 minutes hands-on prep time

MAKES ABOUT 2¾ CUPS; 3 SERVINGS

Each 1-Decadent-Disk serving (heaping ¾ cup) has: 105 calories, 6 g protein, 10 g carbohydrates, 4 g fat, <1 g saturated fat, trace cholesterol, 2 mg fiber, 124 mg sodium

You save: 52 calories, 9 g fat, 4 g saturated fat

Traditional serving: 157 calories, 6 g protein, 8 g carbohydrates, 13 g fat, 5 g saturated fat, 15 mg cholesterol, 2 g fiber, 300 mg sodium

BASIL BUTTERNUT SMASH

One of my commitments to healthy cooking is to transform foods that people might not normally eat into something that is much more familiar. I have a basil mashed potato recipe that's always a huge hit. I love the garlicky flavor and the taste of the fresh basil and Parmesan. In the end, you don't really taste the potatoes much. So I thought these flavors might also work with butternut squash. I was exceptionally pleased with the results, particularly because I'd never been much of a fan of squash. This dish changed my mind.

Please note that butternut squash is often available peeled and cubed in the produce section of major grocery stores. If you opt for that, use only 1 1/2 pounds of the peeled and cubed version in this recipe.

Olive oil spray
2 one-pound butternut squash
2 tablespoons fat-free milk
2 teaspoons light butter
2 tablespoons finely chopped fresh basil
1 1/2 teaspoons grated reduced-fat Parmesan
1 teaspoon minced fresh garlic
Salt and pepper

Preheat the oven to 400°F.

Lightly mist a medium nonstick baking sheet with spray.

Cut the squash in half lengthwise, and then cut the ends off. Use a veggie peeler to peel the skin from the squash. Scrape out the seeds with a spoon. Cut the squash into 1-inch pieces and transfer it to the prepared baking sheet. Bake for 15 minutes. Flip and bake for another 10 to 15 minutes, or until tender throughout.

Combine the milk and butter in a small microwave-safe bowl. Microwave on low until the butter is melted, 30 seconds to 1 minute.

Transfer the squash to a medium mixing bowl and use an electric mixer fitted with beaters to beat on medium speed until smooth. Add the milk mixture, basil, Parmesan, and garlic and continue mixing on low until all of the ingredients are well combined, using a spatula to scrape the bowl from time to time. Season with salt and pepper to taste. Serve immediately.

MAKES ABOUT 2 CUPS; 3 SERVINGS

Each 1-Decadent-Disk serving (heaping 2/3 cup) has: 108 calories, 3 g protein, 24 g carbohydrates, 2 g fat, 1 g saturated fat, 4 mg cholesterol, 4 g fiber, 54 mg sodium

GRILLED CORN ON THE COB

When I was a kid, the only cooked vegetable I would eat was corn on the cob. I wouldn't even eat frozen or canned corn. It had to be on the cob. Quirky, I know. Now I particularly crave corn on the cob in the summer months when sweet corn is so prevalent. Fortunately, this is a really easy recipe that anyone can make, and, unlike many other corn-on-the-cob recipes, it takes only minutes to get the corn on the grill.

You might take special note of the difference in fat and calories in this version versus the traditional one. I was shocked to learn how fattening one ear of corn could possibly be.

4 medium ears fresh corn
2 tablespoons light butter
$^1/_2$ teaspoon seasoned salt, or to taste
3 tablespoons plus 1 teaspoon minced fresh garlic

Preheat a grill to high.

Remove the husks and silks from the corn.

Put the butter, seasoned salt to taste, and garlic in a small microwave-safe bowl. Microwave on high for 30 seconds to 1 minute, or until the butter is melted.

Place one ear of corn in the center of a square of foil large enough to completely cover the corn. Brush a quarter of the butter mixture evenly over the corn, covering all sides. Wrap the foil snugly around the corn. Repeat with the remaining corn and butter mixture.

Lay the wrapped ears side by side, not touching, on the grill. Grill for 20 minutes, rotating every 5 minutes, or until tender. Remove from the grill and carefully remove the foil, being mindful not to burn yourself. Serve immediately.

Can be made in 30 minutes or less / No more than 20 minutes hands-on prep time

MAKES 4 EARS; 4 SERVINGS

Each 1-Decadent-Disk serving (1 ear) has: 103 calories, 3 g protein, 19 g carbohydrates, 2 g fiber, 4 g fat, 2 g saturated fat, 8 mg cholesterol, 206 mg sodium

You save: 184 calories, 20 g fat, 13 g saturated fat

Traditional serving: 287 calories, 3 g protein, 19 g carbohydrates, 24 g fat, 15 g saturated fat, 61 mg cholesterol, 3 g fiber, 1,921 mg sodium

FRIED ZUCCHINI

✦**1**✦

I was recently around a group of true foodies who were resistant to the idea of using garlic powder or reduced-fat Parmesan cheese. And while, in theory, the chef in me totally agrees, in practice, it sometimes just makes sense. But I know, when using these ingredients, I have to be extra careful to create the perfect flavor combinations.

This dish won my foodie friends over. With one bite, they totally loved it.

Olive oil spray (real olive oil, not Pam)
1¹/₂ teaspoons unbleached all-purpose flour
2 tablespoons plain dried bread crumbs
1¹/₂ teaspoons grated reduced-fat Parmesan
1 teaspoon finely chopped fresh parsley
¹/₂ teaspoon garlic powder
¹/₄ teaspoon dried oregano
¹/₈ teaspoon salt
¹/₈ teaspoon black pepper
1 large egg white
2 small zucchini (about 4 ounces each), cut into
     ³/₄-inch rounds (about 12 rounds)
¹/₃ cup Mostly Mom's Marinara Sauce (page 101),
     or your favorite low-fat marinara sauce

Preheat the oven to 425°F.

Mist a medium nonstick baking sheet with spray.

Spoon the flour into a medium shallow bowl.

Put the bread crumbs, Parmesan, parsley, garlic powder, oregano, salt, and pepper in a medium resealable plastic bag.

Use a fork to beat the egg white in a small bowl until bubbly.

Dip both sides of one zucchini round in the flour, and then roll it to coat it completely. Shake off any excess and dip it in the egg to cover it. Let any excess drip off, and then drop the round into the crumb bag and shake gently to coat it. Repeat with each round, and then place them in a single layer, not touching, on the prepared baking sheet.

Lightly mist the tops with spray. Bake for 7 minutes, and then carefully flip them and bake for another 4 to 6 minutes, or until the outsides are golden brown and the insides are tender. Lightly mist the tops with spray.

Meanwhile, just before the zucchini is done, put the marinara sauce in a small microwave-safe bowl. Microwave on low in 30-second intervals until warm. Serve the zucchini immediately with the marinara sauce on the side for dipping.

Can be made in 30 minutes or less / No more than 20 minutes hands-on prep time

---

MAKES ABOUT 12 ROUNDS; 1 SERVING OR 2 PORTIONS

✦**1**✦ Each 1-Decadent-Disk portion (6 pieces with about 3 tablespoons sauce) has: 94 calories, 6 g protein, 16 g carbohydrates, 1 g fat, trace saturated fat, 0 mg cholesterol, 3 g fiber, 361 mg sodium

You save: 79 calories, 11 g fat, 1 g saturated fat

Traditional serving: 173 calories, 5 g protein, 13 g carbohydrates, 12 g fat, 2 g saturated fat, 70 mg cholesterol, 2 g fiber, 400 mg sodium

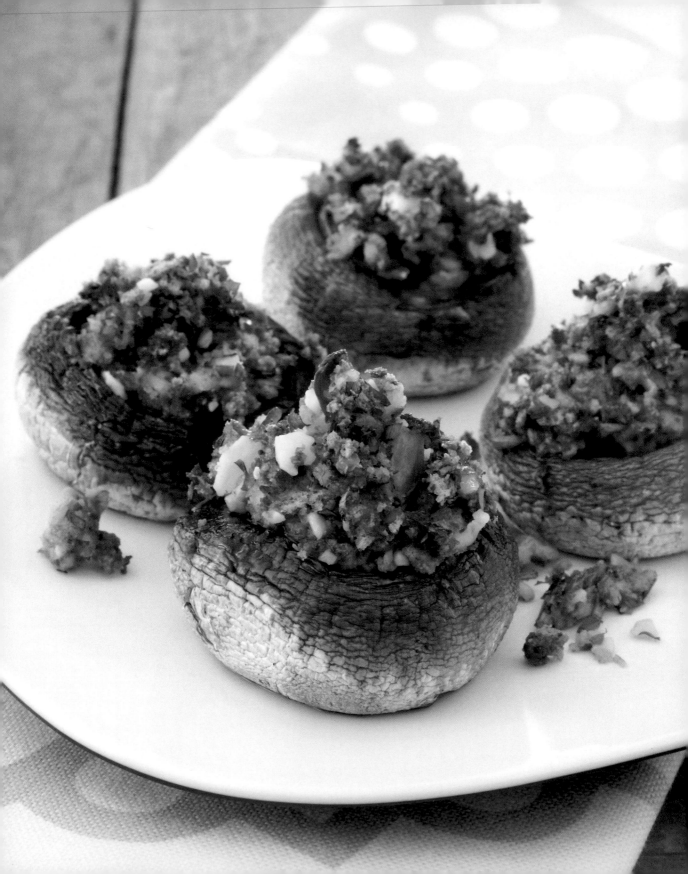

CILANTRO QUESO STUFFED MUSHROOMS

I like to think of Mexican queso as a cross between mozzarella and feta. It's mild like mozzarella, but crumbles like feta. This pale yellow cheese is most often found in U.S. grocery stores in a round block. I've gotten hooked on it in recent years. And there are only about 5 or 6 grams of fat per ounce in the part-skim variety (always buy the one with the least amount of fat that you can find). I often use a touch in salads and here as a twist on an old favorite.

I like spicier food, so I always sprinkle these mushrooms with a salt free Mexican seasoning (see page 17) after they are cooked. Plus, it makes them prettier. If you like milder flavors, feel free to skip it. Whatever you do, don't run the mushrooms under water to clean them. Mushrooms will soak up water, which can kill their flavor and affect the texture. Instead, peel them to remove any dirt or clean them with a damp paper towel.

Olive oil spray
12 medium button mushrooms
2 tablespoons minced fresh garlic
3/4 cup loosely packed fresh cilantro
1 slice whole-wheat bread
3 ounces (about 1/2 cup) crumbled, part-skim queso fresco
1/2 large egg white
1/8 teaspoon salt, plus more to taste
Black pepper
Salt-free Mexican seasoning, optional

Preheat the oven to 400° F. Lightly mist a small nonstick baking sheet with spray.

Clean the mushrooms. Slice the very ends off the stems and discard them. Then pull the remaining stems from the caps, transfer the stems to the bowl of a food processor fitted with a chopping blade, and process until minced. Be careful not to overprocess.

Lightly mist a small nonstick skillet with spray and place it over medium-high heat. Transfer the minced stems to the pan along with the garlic and cook, stirring occasionally, until they are tender and all excess moisture has evaporated, about 5 minutes.

Meanwhile, add the cilantro and bread to the bowl of the food processor and process until minced.

Transfer the mushroom mixture to a medium mixing bowl. Add the bread crumb mixture, queso fresco, and egg white and mix with a wooden spoon until well combined. Season with salt and pepper to taste and Mexican seasoning, if using.

Lightly mist the mushroom caps with spray and sprinkle evenly with salt and pepper to taste. Place them side by side on the baking sheet. Use a small spoon to scoop a heaping mound (about 1 scant tablespoon) of filling atop each cap, dividing the mixture evenly among them. Bake for 10 to 12 minutes, or until the mushrooms are tender and the filling is hot throughout. Serve immediately.

Can be made in 30 minutes or less / No more than 20 minutes hands-on prep time

MAKES 12 MUSHROOMS; 3 SERVINGS

Each 1-Decadent-Disk serving (4 mushrooms) has: 94 calories, 8 g protein, 11 g carbohydrates, 3 g fat, 2 g saturated fat, 9 mg cholesterol, 2 g fiber, 203 mg sodium

ASPARAGUS WITH SHERRY SHALLOT VINAIGRETTE

My friend Cristina makes it very clear that she does not eat low-fat food. When she first met me, she was one of those people who adamantly said that there is no way healthy food tastes good. Though she's beautiful and in great shape, she always cooks with tons of olive oil and lots of butter.

One night she was having a dinner party, and I brought this dish. She went insane over it. She kept saying, "There's no way this dressing is lower-fat." She's since eaten this dish over and over and even served it to her guests.

These days she does concede that certain healthy dishes taste even better than the traditional varieties. But when anyone who is not me says they made something healthy, she still has no desire to try it. So many people feel this way; I hope this book can change the way they think about healthy food.

1¼ pounds medium asparagus spears
1 recipe Sherry Shallot Vinaigrette (recipe follows)

Trim the asparagus by snapping the ends off the stems where they break naturally. Discard the end pieces.

Place a steamer rack in a large pot. Fill the pot with water to just below the rack. Place the pot over high heat and bring the water to a boil. Put in the asparagus, cover, and cook until crisp-tender, 2 to 5 minutes, depending on the thickness of the spears. Transfer the asparagus to a large bowl of ice water. Drain well and dry with paper towels. Return the asparagus to the empty bowl and toss with 1½ tablespoons of Sherry Shallot Vinaigrette. Transfer to a platter or divide among 3 plates. Then drizzle the remaining vinaigrette (about 3½ tablespoons) over the top.

SHERRY SHALLOT VINAIGRETTE

2 tablespoons sherry wine vinegar
1 tablespoon Dijon mustard
1½ teaspoons honey
1 tablespoon extra virgin olive oil
1 tablespoon minced shallots
1 teaspoon minced fresh garlic
1 teaspoon finely chopped fresh tarragon
Salt and pepper

Whisk the vinegar, mustard, and honey in a small bowl. Slowly whisk in the olive oil. Stir in the shallots, garlic, and tarragon. Season with salt and pepper to taste. The vinaigrette can be made up to 5 days in advance and stored in the refrigerator.

Makes about 5 tablespoons
Each tablespoon has: 34 calories, trace protein, 3 g carbohydrates, 3 g fat, trace saturated fat, 0 mg cholesterol, trace fiber, 71 mg sodium

---

Can be made in 30 minutes or less / No more than 20 minutes hands-on prep time

MAKES 3 SERVINGS

Each 1-Decadent-Disk serving (⅓ recipe) has: 97 calories, 3 g protein, 11 g carbohydrates, 5 g fat, <1 g saturated fat, 0 mg cholesterol, 3 g fiber, 118 mg sodium

OVEN-ROASTED BROCCOLI WITH PARMESAN

Broccoli has gotten such a bad rap in the diet world. People are just so sick of eating steamed broccoli. So when I do steam it for recipes like Broccoli Limone (page 179), I add tons of flavor. Here, instead of steaming I roast it with some of my all-time favorite ingredients, garlic and Parmesan, which give it a new life and take eating it from a chore to a delight.

1 pound (about 6^1/$_2$ cups) broccoli florets

2 tablespoons grated reduced-fat Parmesan

1 tablespoon plus 1 teaspoon chopped fresh parsley

1 teaspoon garlic powder

^{1}/$_4$ teaspoon black pepper

Salt

^{1}/$_4$ teaspoon crushed red pepper flakes, optional

1 tablespoon plus 1 teaspoon extra virgin olive oil

Preheat the oven to 425°F.

Trim the broccoli, leaving about ^{1}/$_2$ inch of stem attached to the florets. Toss the broccoli in a large bowl with the Parmesan, parsley, garlic powder, black pepper, and salt to taste. Toss in the red pepper flakes, if using. Drizzle with olive oil and toss again until all of the florets are thoroughly coated.

Transfer to a medium nonstick baking sheet and bake for 10 minutes, and then toss the broccoli again and bake for another 5 to 7 minutes, or until the florets are lightly browned and tender. Serve immediately.

Can be made in 30 minutes or less / No more than 20 minutes hands-on prep time

MAKES 5 CUPS; 4 SERVINGS

Each 1-Decadent-Disk serving (1^1/$_4$ cups) has: 95 calories, 4 g protein, 9 g carbohydrates, 4 g fiber, 6 g fat, <1 g saturated fat, 0 mg cholesterol, 91 mg sodium

You save: 38 calories, 5 g fat, 1 g saturated fat

Traditional serving: 133 calories, 5 g protein, 7 g carbohydrates, 11 g fat, 2 g saturated fat, 4 mg cholesterol, 3 g fiber, 133 mg sodium

SNAP PEA STIR-FRY

Stir-fries, when made without too much oil, are a great answer for those who don't have a lot of time to cook. Whether you're craving chicken and want a hearty dish like a Sweet-and-Sour Chicken Bowl (page 147) or just need a veggie side in a hurry, the prevalence of stir-fry sauces, trimmed and chopped veggies, and bags of frozen veggie assortments makes cooking at home the way to go.

Here the sauce is homemade, but still quick. Just please don't cut corners in this recipe (or any of mine) by using pre-minced garlic. Some pre-minced varieties are packed in oil, which adds unneeded fat and calories (save those extras for another couple of bites of Chocolate Not-Only-in-Your-Dreams Cake, page 210, or one of your other faves from this book). The remainder of it tends to be packed in citric acid, which adds a bitterness and really takes away from that intensely amazing taste. I do, however, recommend buying the peeled cloves to save time.

1 pound sugar snap peas
1 teaspoon extra virgin olive oil
1 tablespoon minced peeled fresh ginger
2 teaspoons minced fresh garlic
1 tablespoon lower-sodium soy sauce
2 teaspoons hoisin sauce
1½ teaspoons rice wine vinegar
1½ teaspoons white or black sesame seeds, optional

Pull off the very ends of the snap peas to trim and remove the strings.

Preheat a large nonstick wok or skillet over medium-high heat. When the wok is hot, put in the olive oil, snap peas, ginger, and garlic. Stirring constantly, cook until the garlic begins to soften, about 1 minute. Next, add the soy sauce, hoisin sauce, and vinegar. Cook until the snap peas are crisp-tender, another 2 to 3 minutes. Remove from the heat and stir in the sesame seeds, if using. Serve immediately.

Can be made in 30 minutes or less / No more than 20 minutes hands-on prep time

MAKES 4 CUPS; 3 SERVINGS

 Each 1-Decadent-Disk serving (1⅓ cups) has: 100 calories, 4 g protein, 15 g carbohydrates, 2 g fat, trace saturated fat, trace cholesterol, 4 g fiber, 257 mg sodium

COLORFUL COLESLAW

1

Last year, I went to my friend Greg's Super Bowl party. He's a great cook and always goes crazy on Super Bowl weekend. He starts the day with his famous Breakfast Ribs in the morning. He then moves on to jambalaya, brats, and by evening, there are "Dessert Ribs." It's one of the few days I indulge in a few bites of everything, because it's all just so insanely good! And it doesn't hurt that he never even lets me help, so I get a true day off.

Last year, the menu also included the most incredible coleslaw I'd ever eaten. I took one bite and was hooked. I started picking it apart and within three days, I created this version that is now my all-time favorite coleslaw recipe. Something about the combo of creamy dressing, fresh herbs, and two varieties of onions had me craving it. Add to that the fact that traditional coleslaw has about 266 calories, 23 grams of fat, 3 grams of saturated fat, and 20 milligrams of cholesterol, and you'll understand why I see this one as 100 percent delicious, and guilt free.

$1/3$ cup light mayonnaise
$1/3$ cup fat-free plain yogurt
2 tablespoons apple cider vinegar
1 tablespoon fat-free milk
2 teaspoons sugar
4 cups packed shredded green cabbage
$3^1/2$ cups packed shredded red cabbage
$1/2$ cup shredded carrots
$1/2$ cup chopped fresh parsley
$1/4$ cup red onion slivers
$1/4$ cup chopped whole green onion
$1/4$ teaspoon salt, or to taste
Black pepper

Whisk the mayonnaise, yogurt, vinegar, milk, and sugar in a large resealable container. Add the green and red cabbage, carrots, parsley, red onion, and green onion. Stir until well combined. Season with salt and pepper to taste. Seal the container and refrigerate for 3 hours to 2 days.

MAKES ABOUT 5$1/4$ CUPS; 6 SERVINGS

1 Each 1-Decadent-Disk serving (heaping $3/4$ cup) has: 92 calories, 3 g protein, 13 g carbohydrates, 4 g fat, trace saturated fat, 4 mg cholesterol, 3 g fiber, 249 mg sodium

You save: 174 calories, 19 g fat, 3 g saturated fat

Traditional serving: 266 calories, 1 g protein, 16 g carbohydrates, 23 g fat, 3 g saturated fat, 20 mg cholesterol, 1 g fiber, 246 mg sodium

WE'VE HEARD IT TIME AND TIME AGAIN: "It's better to eat lots of smaller meals (or snacks) throughout the day than to eat two or three larger meals," as people often do. Yes, it takes a little more time to prepare multiple meals, but that's where you can get creative. I'm a huge fan of eating smaller portions of leftovers as snacks. If you made Chicken Enchilasagna (page 134) for dinner last night, why not heat up a half portion for a snack today? Or if you need more variety, there are hundreds of lower-fat, lower-calorie choices to keep your body fueled throughout the day. I've compiled a few handfuls of my favorites that keep me satisfied. I think you'll like them too.

1 Bite-sized Chili Tostadas

1 **2** Tiny Tacos

3 Buffalo Wing Plate

1 Mediterranean Layer Dip with Toasted Pita Triangles

2 Exotic Tuna Tartare

2 Chicken Satay with Peanut Dipping Sauce

1 Better Bruschetta

1 Bacon Horseradish Dip with Raw Vegetables

2 Dijon Marinated Shrimp

BITE-SIZED CHILI TOSTADAS

⭐

I'd never heard of Frito Pies until earlier this year when I mentioned to my friend Kelly that I was thinking of serving chili on baked tortilla chips for a party. She got all excited and launched into her childhood memories of opening a small bag of Fritos and mounding chili, cheese, and onions right in the bag. In Texas, they apparently do this all the time. It's an awesome concept and, of course, I've done some doctoring of it. Not only does my version save tons of fat and calories, one could even argue that it's taken chili upscale. Either way, I have a feeling that it might get some Texans (and non-Texans) rehooked on this great flavor combination.

10 Tostitos Baked! Scoops
10 teaspoons finely shredded Cabot's 75% Light Cheddar cheese, or your favorite low-fat Cheddar, divided
5 tablespoons Chipotle Chili (without the blue cheese; page 129)
5 teaspoons finely chopped sweet onion, divided

Arrange the Scoops side by side on a plate. Sprinkle 1 teaspoon cheese evenly inside each. Spoon 1^{1}/$_{2}$ teaspoons of hot Chipotle Chili over that, and then sprinkle ^{1}/$_{2}$ teaspoon onions evenly over the top of each. Serve immediately.

MAKES 10 BITE-SIZED TOSTADAS; 1 SERVING OR 2 PORTIONS

⭐ Each 1-Decadent-Disk portion (5 tostadas) has: 101 calories, 9 g protein, 13 g carbohydrates, 2 g fat, trace saturated fat, 9 mg cholesterol, 2 g fiber, 214 mg sodium

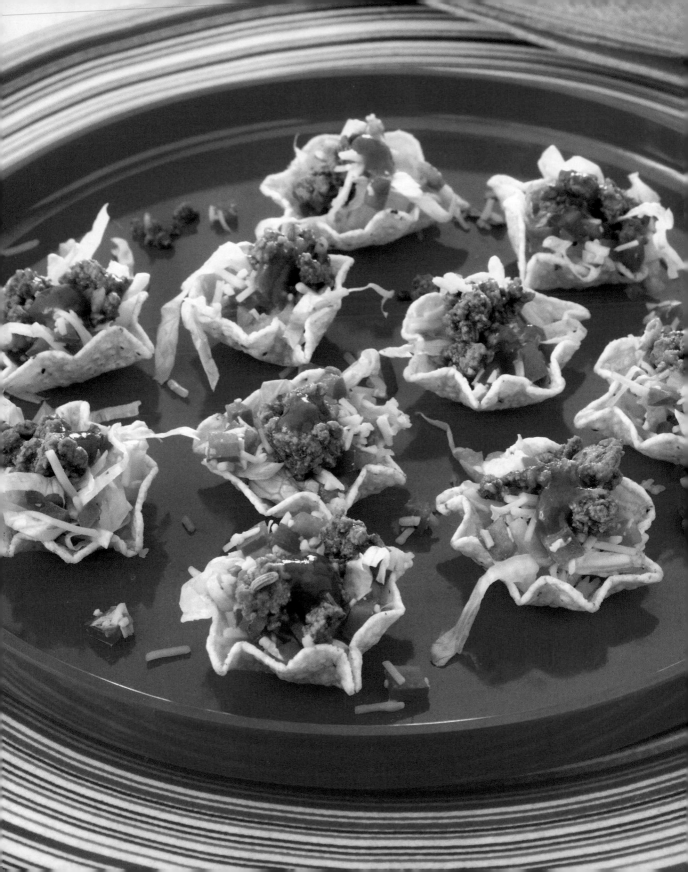

TINY TACOS

1 **2**

These miniaturized versions of tacos are one of my all-time favorite, kid-friendly snacks. When Frito-Lay introduced Baked! Scoops, I was so excited that I instantly went to work on creating dishes to fill these little morsels. I just find them so festive. When I conjured these tacos, I couldn't wait to show them to friends and clients. They're so much fun. Not only can you eat ten of them (how often do you get to eat ten whole anything—outside this book, anyway—when you're eating healthy?) for only 200 calories. Plus the whole family will be excited to dig into your "diet food." And kids will be more than willing to help prepare them.

10 Tostitos Baked! Scoops
1/4 cup finely shredded romaine lettuce
2 tablespoons finely chopped tomatoes
1/2 ounce (about 2 1/2 tablespoons) finely shredded
    Cabot's 75% Light Cheddar cheese, or your
    favorite low-fat Cheddar
1 teaspoon lower-sodium taco seasoning
2 ounces 96% lean ground beef
1 tablespoon mild or hot red taco sauce

Arrange the Scoops side by side on a plate.

Mix the lettuce, tomatoes, and cheese in a medium bowl until well combined. Divide evenly among the Scoops (about 1 1/2 teaspoons per Scoop).

Stir 2 teaspoons water into the taco seasoning in a small bowl until it has no lumps. Set aside.

Preheat a small nonstick skillet over medium-high heat. Put in the beef. Use a wooden spoon to coarsely crumble the meat as it cooks. When the beef is no longer pink, after 1 to 2 minutes, stir in the seasoning mixture. When no liquid remains, after about 1 minute, remove from the heat. Divide the meat evenly among the Scoops, atop the lettuce mixture (about 1 teaspoon in each). Dollop the top of each with taco sauce. Serve immediately.

Can be made in 30 minutes or less / No more than 20 minutes hands-on prep time

MAKES 10 TINY TACOS; 1 SERVING OR 2 PORTIONS

1 Each 1-Decadent-Disk portion (5 tacos) has: 101 calories, 9 g protein, 9 g carbohydrates, 3 g fat, <1 g saturated fat, 18 mg cholesterol, <1 g fiber, 223 mg sodium

2 Each 2-Decadent-Disk serving (10 tacos) has: 202 calories, 17 g protein, 19 g carbohydrates, 6 g fat, 2 g saturated fat, 35 mg cholesterol, 2 g fiber, 446 mg sodium

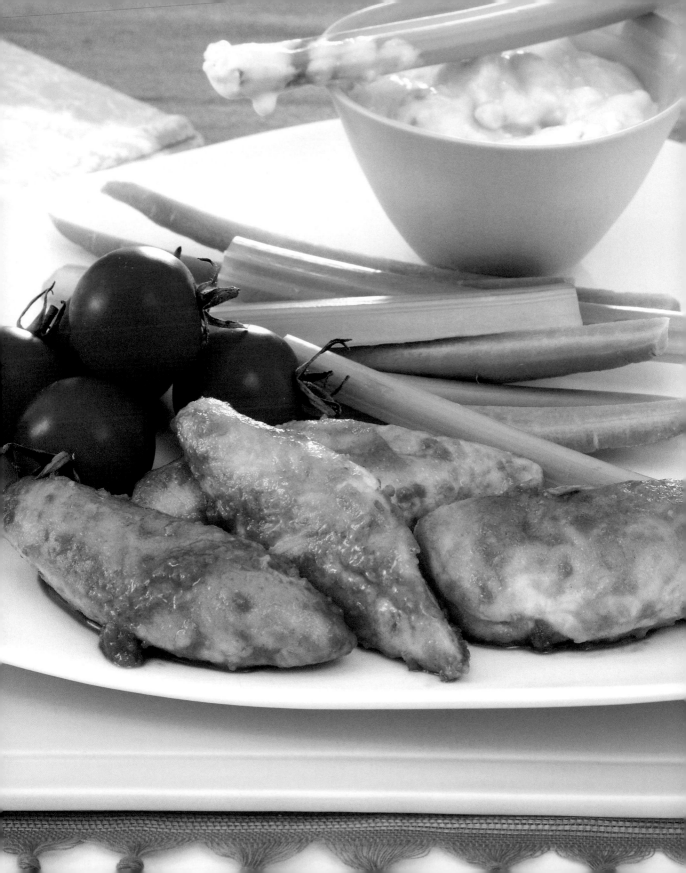

BUFFALO WING PLATE

3

This dish is one of my favorite snack items. Not only does it help me get enough veggies in my diet, the plate contains a lot of food with tons of flavor, particularly for less than 300 calories. Plus, it feels so off-limits, which, for me, always adds to the enjoyment. It seems like you're getting away with something, since you're eating a dish that you know is just insanely out of control in fat and calories when you order it at the local pub. I often serve this plate as a starter when I have my girlfriends over to watch our favorite reality TV shows.

2¹/₂ tablespoons Blue Cheese Dressing (recipe follows)
4 Boneless Buffalo Strips (recipe follows)
1 medium stalk celery, cut into sticks
1 medium carrot, cut into sticks
6 cherry tomatoes

Spoon the dressing into a small dipping bowl. Arrange the Boneless Buffalo Strips on a plate with the celery, carrots, tomatoes, and dressing. Serve immediately.

BONELESS BUFFALO STRIPS

I generally use chicken tenderloins, as opposed to chicken breasts, for this dish because it saves time. But if the tenderloins are significantly more expensive at your grocery store and you want to save money, you can use chicken breasts. You'll need about four 4-ounce chicken breasts. Just pound them to an even ¹/₄-inch thickness using the flat side of a meat mallet, and then cut each on a diagonal into four equal strips.

When you're cooking the chicken, it's very important to use a large pan or work in batches. The strips should be cooked in a single layer, not touching. The pan should also be very hot. If cooked as described, the strips will be lightly golden on the outside and very tender on the inside. If not, the moisture released from the chicken will steam it, preventing the chicken from browning and cooking properly.

1¹/₂ tablespoons unbleached all-purpose flour
¹/₄ teaspoon garlic powder
¹/₄ teaspoon salt   *(continued)*

Can be made in 30 minutes or less

MAKES 1 SERVING

3 Each 3-Decadent-Disk serving has: 293 calories, 32 g protein, 18 g carbohydrates, 10 g fat, 4 g saturated fat, 83 mg cholesterol, 4 g fiber, 782 mg sodium

You save: 302 calories, 38 g fat, 13 g saturated fat

Traditional serving: 595 calories, 31 g protein, 15 g carbohydrates, 48 g fat, 17 g saturated fat, 138 mg cholesterol, 4 g fiber, 1,429 mg sodium

16 chicken tenderloins (about 1 pound), trimmed
   of tendons
Olive oil spray
2 tablespoons light butter (stick, not tub)
1¹/₂ tablespoons hot sauce (a thick one like
   Frank's), plus more to taste

Mix the flour, garlic powder, and salt in a
medium shallow bowl until well combined.

Dip one chicken strip at time into the flour
mixture and turn it to coat completely. Then
shake off any excess flour. Transfer the strip to
a plate. Repeat with the remaining strips,
placing them side by side on the plate until
they are all coated.

Place a large nonstick skillet over high heat.
When the skillet is hot, lightly mist it with spray
and add the chicken strips side by side, not
touching, in a single layer (work in batches, if
necessary). Cook until lightly browned on the
outside and no longer pink inside, 2 to
3 minutes per side.

Meanwhile, place a small, nonstick skillet
over low heat and add the butter and hot
sauce. Heat, stirring constantly, until the butter
is just melted, being careful not to scorch it.
Immediately remove from the heat, add the
chicken strips, and toss to coat completely.
Add more hot sauce, if desired. Let stand in
the pan for 5 minutes, and then toss again (the
sauce will stick better after resting) and serve
immediately.

Makes 16 strips; 4 servings
Each 4-strip serving has: 162 calories, 27 g protein,
3 g carbohydrates, 5 g fat, 2 g saturated fat,
73 mg cholesterol, trace fiber, 427 mg sodium

BLUE CHEESE DRESSING

I love this dressing. When it's first made it's rich
and creamy just like the fatty versions, and it's
completely aftertaste free, unlike many of the
lower-fat ones. Just note that you shouldn't
make this far in advance of serving it. It will
become thinner over time, so it's best served
within a couple of hours.

¹/₄ cup light mayonnaise
3 tablespoons fat-free sour cream
3 tablespoons low-fat buttermilk
¹/₂ teaspoon hot sauce
¹/₂ teaspoon cider vinegar
¹/₂ cup crumbled reduced-fat blue cheese

Whisk the mayonnaise, sour cream, buttermilk,
hot sauce, and vinegar in a medium resealable
container until smooth and well combined. Stir
in the blue cheese until well combined. Seal
the container and refrigerate for at least 1 hour.

Makes about ³/₄ cup plus 1 tablespoon
Two tablespoons have: 62 calories, 2 g protein,
2 g carbohydrates, 4 g fat, 1 g saturated fat,
8 mg cholesterol, 206 mg sodium
You save: 102 calories, 13 g fat, 3 g saturated fat,
46 mg sodium
Traditional 2 tablespoons: 164 calories, 1 g protein,
2 g carbohydrates, 17 g fat, 4 g saturated fat,
17 mg cholesterol, trace fiber, 149 mg sodium

MEDITERRANEAN LAYER DIP WITH TOASTED PITA TRIANGLES

When you hear "Seven Layer Dip," you probably immediately think of that scrumptious Mexican dip that is often served at parties along with mounds of tortilla chips. Well, here's a Mediterranean spin that's not only just as tasty, it's much lighter than the dip you are used to. It also combines tons of flavors and fresh veggies in a pretty and festive way. Three tablespoons of the dip on its own have only 41 calories and 2 grams of fat.

When buying the garlic hummus for this dip (and always), be sure to read labels. Though many are relatively low in fat, every once in a while you may find one brand that is significantly higher. I used a very popular brand that has 3 grams of fat per 2-tablespoon serving when writing this recipe. Make sure to find one that is in that ballpark, if at all possible.

1 cup garlic-flavored hummus
$1/2$ cup fat-free plain yogurt
$1/4$ teaspoon ground cumin
$1/2$ teaspoon finely chopped fresh mint
$1^1/3$ cups seeded and finely chopped cucumbers (see page 21)
$1^1/3$ cups seeded and finely chopped Roma tomatoes (see page 21)

2 teaspoons finely chopped fresh parsley
1 teaspoon fresh lemon juice
1 teaspoon minced fresh garlic
Pinch of salt
$1/4$ cup finely chopped red onion
3 ounces reduced-fat feta cheese, crumbled
2 tablespoons chopped Kalamata olives (about 8 olives)
6 (About $6^1/2$-inch-diameter) whole-wheat pita circles, lightly toasted and cut into wedges

Spoon the hummus into a 6-cup glass bowl. Use a spatula to spread it evenly to make one layer.

Mix the yogurt with the cumin and mint in a small bowl. Pour the yogurt mixture evenly over the hummus and smooth it with the back of a spoon to form a second layer. Sprinkle the cucumbers evenly over the top.

Mix the tomatoes, parsley, lemon juice, garlic, and salt in a medium bowl. Sprinkle the tomato mixture over the cucumbers, followed by the onion, feta, then the olives.

Cover with plastic wrap and refrigerate for 1 to 6 hours. Serve with pita triangles for dipping.

MAKES ABOUT $3^1/2$ CUPS DIP; ABOUT 18 SERVINGS

Each 1-Decadent-Disk serving ($1/3$ pita circle with 3 tablespoons dip) has: 97 calories, 5 g protein, 15 g carbohydrates, 3 g fat, <1 g saturated fat, 2 mg cholesterol, 3 g fiber, 270 mg sodium

EXOTIC TUNA TARTARE

2

I was recently judging a cooking competition for Chefs.com. They flew me out to San Francisco, where I had time to check out the city. In my case, that means check out some restaurants. I happened upon this little hole in the wall that had a review of their tuna tartare on the door. Since I love tartare, I decided to grab a seat at the bar and give it a try.

I took a couple of bites as I chatted with a bartender who seemed very knowledgeable about the menu. Just as I was thinking the dish needed salt, he said, "Do you think it has enough salt?" He brought me a tiny container of an exotic sea salt with the tiniest little spoon I'd ever seen and said, "It's amazing how salt makes such a difference." I added just a touch and he was right. It made all of the difference in the world.

So here's a spin on that version. Though I don't expect you to have exotic sea salt, any sea salt will do, and makes an amazing enhancement to this dish, which is probably a touch different than any tartare you've ever had. Just note that if you're not serving it immediately after preparing it, you should omit the lemon juice until just before serving or the juice will start to "cook" the tuna and it will turn color slightly.

If you've never bought fish to eat raw before, there's no need to be intimidated. You simply need to consider a few things. First, never eat raw fish that is not labeled "sushi grade" or "sashimi grade." Then, look carefully at the color. Ahi should be bright red. It could be a lighter red or a deep red, but either way, it should be bright, not dull. Then look carefully at the edges. They should be the same bright shade as the middle. If it's not or the edges are even slightly browned, don't buy it. And it shouldn't smell fishy.

5 ounces sashimi- or sushi-grade ahi tuna, coarsely chopped
1 teaspoon fresh lemon juice
$^1/_2$ teaspoon toasted sesame oil (see page 18)
$^1/_2$ teaspoon extremely finely slivered fresh basil (see page 20)
$^1/_2$ teaspoon extremely finely slivered fresh mint
$^1/_4$ teaspoon seeded and minced green jalapeño pepper
$^1/_4$ teaspoon minced fresh garlic
$^1/_8$ teaspoon hot sesame oil
$^1/_8$ teaspoon sea salt, or to taste

Combine the ahi, lemon juice, toasted sesame oil, basil, mint, jalapeño, garlic, and hot sesame oil in a small soup bowl. Mix until just combined. Season with salt to taste. Transfer to a martini glass, if desired, and serve immediately.

Can be made in 30 minutes or less / No more than 20 minutes hands-on prep time

MAKES 1 SERVING

2 Each 2-Decadent-Disk serving has: 207 calories, 35 g protein, <1 g carbohydrates, 6 g fat, trace saturated fat, 0 mg cholesterol, trace fiber, 295 mg sodium

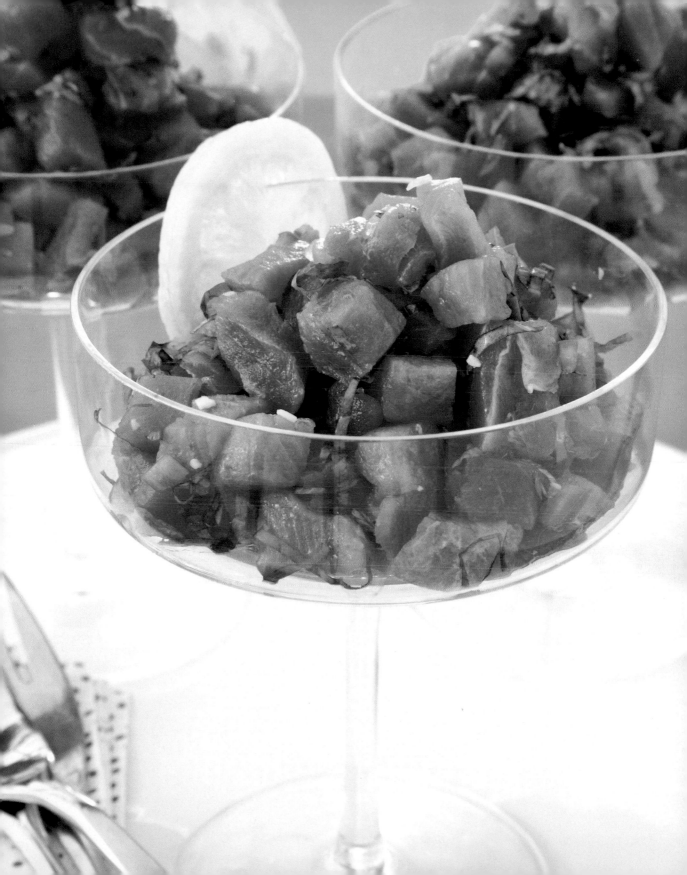

CHICKEN SATAY WITH PEANUT DIPPING SAUCE

2

People often ask my strategy for eating at cocktail parties or weddings, because so often all of the foods are deep-fried or just fat laden. Admittedly, it can be tough, especially at weddings when, without fail, you're always eating hours after you expected and you're starved by the time they start passing the appetizers. So my strategy is always: eat first.

I never go to cocktail parties very hungry, because though most of us could easily eat ten to fifteen of those bite-sized appetizers, less than half that number tend to have the caloric equivalent of what we should be eating at a meal. Add the fact that you're likely to be having a cocktail (or three) and you can set your healthy eating plan way back.

So I eat a small meal at home and then I enjoy a few things at the event for a treat and as part of being social. When I do look around for something to eat, I usually head toward whatever lean protein is being offered. It's often chicken satay here in Los Angeles, and I've really come to love it. When I'm out, however, I rarely eat the dipping sauce because that can be extremely fattening, too. Here's a version that you can enjoy guilt free. Note that the chicken is quite tasty on its own, so if you want to save some time (and calories) you can skip the sauce completely. Three pieces of chicken without the sauce have only 154 calories and less than 3 grams of fat.

2 tablespoons light soy sauce
2 tablespoons sake
2 tablespoons fresh lime juice
2 tablespoons honey
1 tablespoon toasted sesame oil
2 tablespoon minced peeled fresh ginger
2 tablespoons minced fresh garlic
$^1/_2$ teaspoon curry powder
1 pound boneless, skinless chicken breasts, visible fat removed
12 wooden skewers, soaked in water for at least 30 minutes, or metal skewers
4 tablespoons Peanut Dipping Sauce (recipe follows)

MAKES 12 SKEWERS; 4 SERVINGS

2 Each 2-Decadent-Disk serving (3 skewers with 1 tablespoon sauce) has: 201 calories, 28 g protein, 10 g carbohydrates, 5 g fat, 1 g saturated fat, 66 mg cholesterol, 1 g fiber, 261 mg sodium

You save: 190 calories, 20 g fat, 8 g saturated fat

Traditional serving: 391 calories, 33 g protein, 9 g carbohydrates, 25 g fat, 9 g saturated fat, 66 mg cholesterol, 2 g fiber, 315 mg sodium

Whisk the soy sauce, sake, lime juice, honey, sesame oil, ginger, garlic, and curry powder in a medium resealable container.

Place the chicken breasts between two sheets of plastic wrap or wax paper on a flat work surface. Use the flat side of a meat mallet to pound them to an even $\frac{1}{3}$-inch thickness. Cut them into 12 relatively even strips. Add the strips to the marinade and stir to coat thoroughly. Seal the container and refrigerate for at least 6 hours or overnight.

Preheat a grill to high heat.

Remove the chicken pieces from the marinade and let the excess drip off. Carefully thread each chicken piece onto a skewer, working the skewer in and out of the meat, through the center of the piece, so that it stays secure during grilling. Discard the remaining marinade. Grill for 2 to 3 minutes per side, or until the chicken is no longer pink inside. Serve immediately with Peanut Dipping Sauce.

PEANUT DIPPING SAUCE

Olive oil spray
2 garlic cloves, minced (about 1 tablespoon)
2 teaspoons minced onion
3 tablespoons light coconut milk (see page 16)
$\frac{1}{4}$ cup low-sodium chicken broth
2 tablespoons molasses
1 tablespoon light soy sauce
$1\frac{1}{2}$ teaspoons curry powder
$\frac{1}{4}$ teaspoon chili powder
$\frac{1}{4}$ cup reduced-fat peanut butter

Lightly mist a small nonstick saucepan with spray and place it over medium heat. Add the garlic and onion and cook until the garlic and onion begin to soften and become very fragrant, about 2 minutes.

Add the coconut milk, broth, molasses, soy sauce, curry powder, and chili powder. Slowly bring to a boil, then lower the heat and simmer, stirring occasionally, until slightly thickened, about 5 minutes.

Remove from the heat. Slowly whisk in the peanut butter until well incorporated. Transfer to a serving bowl.

Makes a scant $\frac{3}{4}$ cup
Each tablespoon has: 47 calories, 2 g protein, 6 g carbohydrates, 2 g fat, <1 g saturated fat, 0 mg cholesterol, trace fiber, 98 mg sodium

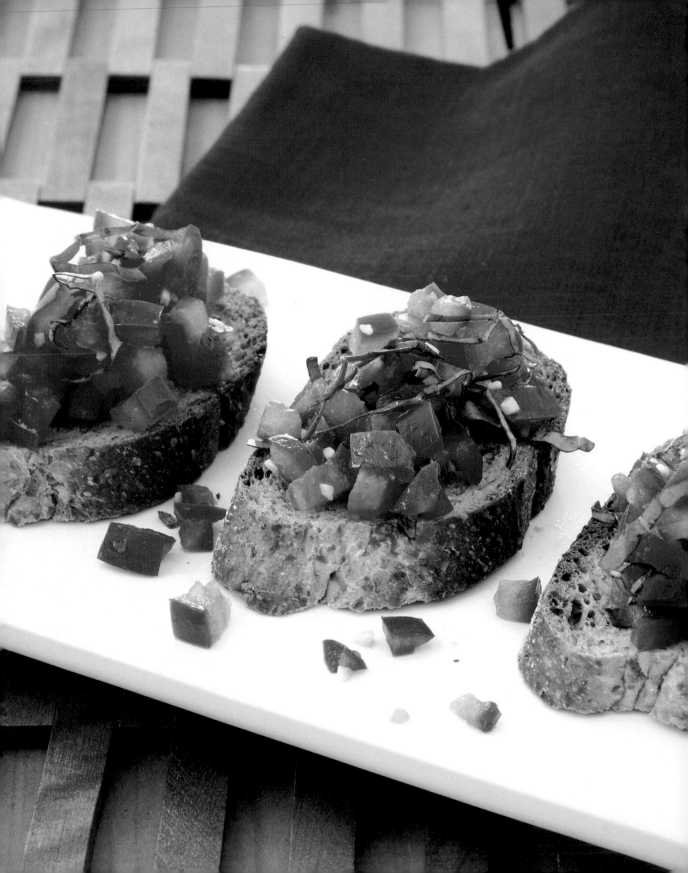

BETTER BRUSCHETTA

I've always loved bruschetta, but I rarely ate it because it can be so fattening. Often the bread is spread with an enormous amount of butter or olive oil, which is really disappointing because by the time you add plenty of fresh tomatoes with the garlic and fresh basil, you really can't tell the difference. And most bruschetta topping has way more oil than necessary. True, olive oil does have "good fat," and you do need some fat in your diet. But people often think they can consume a lot of olive oil without any consequence just because it's "good" fat. To that, I always say, "It's good for your heart, and bad for your hips."

One tablespoon of olive oil has 126 calories and 14 grams of fat. Quickly flipping through this book, you can see the enormous number of satisfying options you have to spend 100 calories on. Do you really want to have a couple of tablespoons of olive oil instead of a whole Chocolate Not-Only-in-Your-Dreams Cake (page 210) or even one tablespoon instead of five Tiny Tacos (page 193)? If you look at it that way, it kind of puts things in perspective, don't you think?

One 2-ounce piece (5 to 6 inches) of a thin
    multigrain or whole-wheat French baguette
2 large garlic cloves, cut in half
6 tablespoons Bruschetta Topping (page 140)

Preheat the oven to 350°F.

Cut the baguette into 6 slices (about $^3/_4$ inch thick) on a diagonal. Place them side by side on a nonstick baking sheet and rub one side of each slice with a cut side of the garlic. Bake for 5 to 8 minutes, until the bread is lightly toasted. Remove from the oven. Top each slice with 1 tablespoon Bruschetta Topping and serve immediately.

Can be made in 30 minutes or less / No more than 20 minutes hands-on prep time

MAKES 6 PIECES; 2 SERVINGS

Each 1-Decadent-Disk serving (3 pieces) has: 108 calories, 3 g protein, 16 g carbohydrates, 3 g fat, trace saturated fat, 0 mg cholesterol, 2 g fiber, 229 mg sodium

BACON HORSERADISH DIP WITH RAW VEGETABLES

I helped cast the first season of *Top Chef* on Bravo and was then asked to be a contestant; I've been addicted to the show ever since. I opted not to be on the show, because the contestants have such a different style of cooking than I do. I like to appeal more to the mainstream, with easily accessible ingredients, and I veer toward mastering comfort foods (plus my foods are much healthier, for the most part).

But I totally admire what the chefs do, and their breadth of knowledge is nothing to scoff at. The other night, I was watching an episode and Ted Allen at the judge's table said it's smart to wrap bacon around shrimp—in America, add bacon to anything and people will eat it.

I chuckled because when my friends and I gathered to come up with the recipe list for this book with the intent of making sure I deliver on "most decadent," people suggested dish after dish with bacon in it. And there are a lot in here (though there were almost even more). Here is one of the recipes that just had to stay, as everyone agreed it is one of the most common decadent dips around.

Feel free to add plenty of horseradish to this if you like it. I always add more, but wanted to make sure it appealed to even milder palates. One tablespoon of horseradish has only 7 calories and less than 1 gram of fat. Also, whatever you do, especially if you are using more, make sure to drain the horseradish well to ensure a creamy dip.

3 tablespoons Bacon Horseradish Dip (recipe follows)
$^1/_3$ cup baby carrots or carrot sticks
$^1/_2$ cup celery sticks
$^1/_2$ cup steamed and chilled broccoli florets

Put the dip in a miniature bowl. Place the bowl on a plate along with the carrots, celery, and broccoli and serve immediately.

BACON HORSERADISH DIP WITH SOURDOUGH WHEAT BREAD CUBES

$^1/_4$ cup Bacon Horseradish Dip (recipe follows)
$1^1/_2$ ounces wheat sourdough bread, cut into bite-sized cubes

Put the dip in a miniature bowl. Place the bowl on a plate along with the bread cubes and serve immediately.

MAKES 1 SERVING
Each 2-Decadent-Disk serving has: 195 calories, 7 g protein, 26 g carbohydrates, 6 g fat, 3 g saturated fat, 22 mg cholesterol, 3 g fiber, 401 mg sodium

No more than 20 minutes hands-on prep time

MAKES 1 SERVING
 Each 1-Decadent-Disk serving has: 106 calories, 5 g protein, 14 g carbohydrates, 4 g fat, 3 g saturated fat, 18 mg cholesterol, 3 g fiber, 256 mg sodium

BACON HORSERADISH DIP

6 slices center-cut bacon, cut in half
¹/₄ cup bottled horseradish, plus more to taste
1 cup light sour cream
¹/₃ cup finely chopped whole green onion

Place the bacon strips side by side in a large nonstick skillet over medium-high heat. Cook until crispy, 3 to 5 minutes per side. Pour the bacon, along with the grease, into a small bowl.

Meanwhile, spoon the horseradish into a fine strainer. Lightly press and stir it with a spoon to drain it. Continue until all excess moisture is removed. Transfer the drained horseradish to a small mixing bowl. Add the sour cream and green onion.

Spoon the bacon from the grease, reserving the grease, and crumble or finely chop it. Stir all but 1 teaspoon of the bacon into the mixture along with 1¹/₂ tablespoons of the reserved bacon grease until well combined. Season with more horseradish, if desired. Cover and refrigerate for at least 1 hour. Stir, and then top with the remaining bacon. Serve immediately.

Makes about 1¹/₃ cups; 11 servings
Each 2-tablespoon serving has: 41 calories, 2 g protein, 4 g carbohydrates, 3 g fat, 2 g saturated fat, 11 mg cholesterol, trace fiber, 107 mg sodium

You save: 97 calories, 12 g fat, 3 g saturated fat

Traditional serving: 138 calories, 2 g protein, 2 g carbohydrates, 11 g fat, 5 g saturated fat, 19 mg cholesterol, trace fiber, 114 mg sodium

DIJON MARINATED SHRIMP

2

One of my local grocery stores has a version of this dish in their deli case. They use extra-jumbo prawns and they're just dripping with this wonderful sauce. I rarely eat them—in addition to being very fattening, they cost $29.99 per pound—but every time I go to buy my deli meats, I see them and *think* about eating them. Finally, I went home and made my own version, so I could stop feeling mildly tortured (okay, I'm exaggerating, but I did want them). I never even flinch at the ones at the store anymore. Why would I, when these are much healthier and I save more than $20 per pound by making them myself?

1^{1}/$_{3}$ pounds large (about 21–25 count) shrimp, unpeeled

3^{1}/$_{2}$ tablespoons Sherry Shallot Vinaigrette (page 186)

1 tablespoon Dijon mustard

1 tablespoon finely chopped fresh flat-leaf parsley

1 teaspoon chopped fresh tarragon

4 butter lettuce leaves, optional

Put a bowl of ice water in the sink. Bring a medium pot of salted water to a boil. Add the shrimp and cook for 1 to 2 minutes, until the outsides turn pink and they are cooked through.

Drain the shrimp and transfer immediately to the bowl of ice water. Drain again. Peel them, leaving the tail and first segment intact. Place the shrimp in a large resealable plastic container.

Whisk the Sherry Shallot Vinaigrette, mustard, parsley, and tarragon in a small bowl. Pour the dressing over the shrimp and toss until well coated. Seal the container and refrigerate for 1 hour to 1 day. Toss again, and then serve chilled divided among 4 martini glasses or 4 plates, each lined with a lettuce leaf, if desired.

No more than 20 minutes hands-on prep time

MAKES 4 SERVINGS

2 Each 2-Decadent-Disk serving (^{1}/$_{4}$ recipe) has: 190 calories, 31 g protein, 4 g carbohydrates, 5 g fat, trace saturated fat, 229 mg cholesterol, trace fiber, 334 mg sodium

You save: 74 calories, 7 g fat, 1 g saturated fat

Traditional serving: 264 calories, 36 g protein, 2 g carbohydrates, 12 g fat, 2 g saturated fat, 330 mg cholesterol, trace fiber, 381 mg sodium

AAAAAH, DESSERT . . . MY FAVORITE. What can I say? If it were an option, I would have put this chapter first. But that could be weird, since this is a "diet" book and you really do need to get your veggies before dessert. Darn!

I think my love for dessert stems back to my childhood. I was never a huge fan of veggies, and I wasn't allowed to have dessert if I didn't eat all of my veggies . . . except on Friday nights. I think that's part of the reason that, by the time I got to high school and my mom lightened up on the food rules, I stayed home and baked instead of going to the school dances. I was like a Pavlovian puppy programmed to get my desserts on Fridays. Then I spent years making up for all of those Saturdays through Thursdays when I just wasn't allowed to have any (I think I'm subconsciously still making up for them).

You'll notice that I use a lot of whole-grain oat flour in this chapter along with brown sugar and lower-fat ingredients. Because I do love dessert so much, a lot of TLC goes into all of my desserts. My goal is always to bring you the best, most satisfying taste with as much fiber and as little sugar as possible. Whether you don't eat white sugar at all or you are just trying to make subtle (in terms of taste) but major (in terms of health) changes, I'm sure you'll love the desserts in this chapter as much as I do!

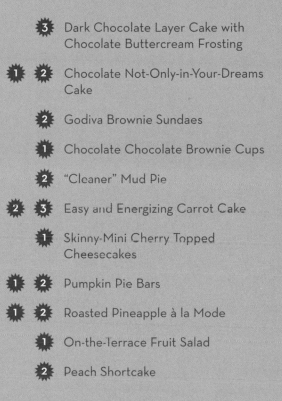

3 Dark Chocolate Layer Cake with Chocolate Buttercream Frosting

1 2 Chocolate Not-Only-in-Your-Dreams Cake

2 Godiva Brownie Sundaes

1 Chocolate Chocolate Brownie Cups

2 "Cleaner" Mud Pie

2 3 Easy and Energizing Carrot Cake

1 Skinny-Mini Cherry Topped Cheesecakes

1 2 Pumpkin Pie Bars

1 2 Roasted Pineapple à la Mode

1 On-the-Terrace Fruit Salad

2 Peach Shortcake

DARK CHOCOLATE LAYER CAKE WITH CHOCOLATE BUTTERCREAM FROSTING

When my first cookbook, *Fast Food Fix*, came out, reporters were constantly trying to get me to admit that I still have a secret fast-food longing. They would say, "Come on, you *must* cheat from time to time with the real deal." But the truth was that I just didn't and I still don't. Once I re-created those flavors, the cravings went away completely.

They never believed me or backed down until I confessed that I have yet to win the war with my cravings for fudge cake. I just love it and I could definitely indulge constantly.

This recipe is a little homage, of sorts, to my love for rich chocolate layer cake—the food that is still my joy and my nemesis, of sorts. Thus the reason it made the cover of this book.

But the good news is, knowing that I can have it whenever I want takes away the obsession I used to have with it. Now, when I do indulge, I truly enjoy every last bite and walk away without a twinge of guilt, particularly because this one is even made with whole-grain flour. The fiber helps fill me up so I don't start looking for another treat right after I'm finished.

Butter-flavored cooking spray
1½ cups whole-grain oat flour (see page 17)
1 cup unsweetened cocoa powder
1 teaspoon baking powder
1 teaspoon baking soda
¼ teaspoon very finely ground espresso beans
¾ teaspoon salt
1 cup low-fat buttermilk
1 teaspoon white vinegar
2 teaspoons vanilla extract
4 large egg whites
2 cups dark or light brown sugar (not packed)
1 cup fat-free, artificially sweetened vanilla yogurt
1 recipe Chocolate Buttercream Frosting (recipe follows)

Preheat the oven to 350°F.

Cut two 9-inch circles of parchment to line the bottoms of two 9-inch nonstick cake pans (trace the pans for ease). Lay the parchment in the pans. Lightly mist the papers and the sides of the pans with spray.

Sift together the flour, cocoa powder, baking powder, baking soda, espresso, and salt in a medium mixing bowl.

Use a sturdy whisk (or an electric mixer, but be careful not to overmix) to mix the buttermilk, vinegar, and vanilla in a large mixing bowl until well combined. Whisk in the egg whites, brown sugar, and yogurt and continue mixing until blended. Gradually stir in the dry

---

MAKES 1 LAYER CAKE; 14 SERVINGS

Each 3-Decadent-Disk serving (1 slice) has: 294 calories, 6 g protein, 59 g carbohydrates, 6 g fat, 3 g saturated fat, 11 mg cholesterol, 4 g fiber, 384 mg sodium

You save: 261 calories, 27 g fat, 17 g saturated fat

Traditional serving: 555 calories, 7 g protein, 65 g carbohydrates, 33 g fat, 20 g saturated fat, 124 mg cholesterol, 4 g fiber, 199 mg sodium

ingredients until just smooth. Divide the batter evenly among the pans. Bake for 16 to 18 minutes, or until a toothpick inserted in the center comes out dry (a few crumbs are okay).

Cool the cakes side by side on a wire cooling rack in the pans for 10 minutes. Then carefully flip the cakes onto the rack. If the cakes stick to the sides of the pans, gently run a butter knife around the rims of the pans to loosen them.

Meanwhile, prepare the Chocolate Buttercream Frosting.

When the cakes are completely cool, place one cake, flat side down, on a platter. Spread $^3/_4$ cup frosting over the top of the cake. Top it with the second cake, flat side down. Spread the remaining frosting evenly over the top and sides of the cake. Slice the cake into 14 equal wedges. Serve immediately, or refrigerate in an airtight container for up to 3 days.

CHOCOLATE BUTTERCREAM FROSTING

I'm an icing girl. When I order a piece of cake in a restaurant these days, I tend to eat a bite or two of the cake with the icing, then a few bites of the icing, and that's it. (And I'm able to stop there only because I know I can make a much less fattening one whenever I want that I'll enjoy more.) So I don't skimp on this icing.

True, it's not exactly mounded on this cake. But I once saw an episode of a healthy cooking show where the host was trying to spread such

a ridiculously small amount of icing over a cake that the cake kept tearing. Finally, they cut away and he pulled out another cake with the thinnest layer of icing you've ever seen and said, "Well, this isn't a cake decorating show, so I have a finished one here." I couldn't believe it. I couldn't watch the show anymore. To me, it's blasphemy to serve a cake with so little icing. Okay, I'm exaggerating, but rest assured, that is not the case here.

$^1/_4$ cup plus 2 tablespoons light butter (stick, not tub), room temperature
$^1/_4$ cup plus 2 tablespoons light cream cheese, room temperature
2 teaspoons vanilla extract
Pinch of salt
$2^3/_4$ cups powdered sugar
$^1/_2$ cup unsweetened cocoa powder
$1^1/_2$ teaspoons fat-free milk

Add the butter, cream cheese, vanilla, and salt to a large mixing bowl. Use an electric mixer fitted with beaters to beat on high speed until smooth. Add half of the powdered sugar. Beat on low speed until well combined. Beat in the remaining powdered sugar and the cocoa powder until combined. Add the milk and beat on high speed until fluffy. Tightly cover the bowl of frosting with plastic wrap until the cakes are cooled (do not refrigerate it before icing the cake).

Makes 2$^1/_4$ cups

CHOCOLATE NOT-ONLY-IN-YOUR-DREAMS CAKE
1 **2**

I dreamed about eating a cake like this for years (both in my sleep and just rapid-fire thoughts during the day). I'm serious. I'm one of those "There's no such thing as chocolate cake that's too rich" types. I was dieting, but I would have to "cheat" with chocolate from time to time just to keep my sanity.

And then came this cake. It's as rich as they come and I love it more than any other flourless chocolate espresso cake I've had. Plus, it packs six grams of fiber, so it really is guilt free!

If you really want to impress your friends, store some, unbaked, in the ramekins in an airtight container in your freezer. When you need a no-fuss dessert, pop them in the water bath and bake them 30 to 32 minutes.

Butter-flavored cooking spray
$^1/_4$ cup unsweetened applesauce
1 teaspoon vanilla extract
4 large egg whites
1 cup dark or light brown sugar (not packed)
$^3/_4$ cup unsweetened cocoa powder
$^1/_4$ teaspoon very finely ground espresso beans
$^1/_2$ teaspoon salt
$^1/_2$ teaspoon powdered sugar
4 raspberries, optional
Four $3^1/_2$-inch-diameter ramekins

Preheat the oven to 350°F.

Generously mist four $3^1/_2$-inch-diameter ramekins with spray. Place them side by side in an 8 X 8-inch baking pan. Add water to the pan until it reaches halfway to the top of the ramekins.

Use a sturdy whisk or spatula to mix the applesauce, vanilla, egg whites, and brown sugar in a large mixing bowl until well combined. Add the cocoa powder, espresso, and salt. Stir until just combined and no lumps remain. Divide evenly among the ramekins (each ramekin will be about two-thirds full).

Bake for 21 to 24 minutes, until the tops look silky and puff slightly and a toothpick inserted in the center comes out a bit wet. Remove from the oven and carefully transfer the rame-kins from the water bath to a cooling rack. Cool for 5 to 10 minutes. Then invert each ramekin onto a dessert plate. Let stand for 1 minute, and then slowly lift off the ramekin (the cakes should come out on their own, but if they don't, run a knife around the edge of the cakes to loosen them). Cool for another 5 to 10 minutes. Use a fine sieve to evenly dust each cake with a light sprinkling of powdered sugar. Place one raspberry on the center of each cake, if using. Serve immediately.

No more than 20 minutes hands-on prep time

MAKES 4 CAKES; 4 SERVINGS OR 8 PORTIONS

1 Each 1-Decadent-Disk portion ($^1/_2$ cake) has: 101 calories, 3 g protein, 23 g carbohydrates, 1 g fat, <1 g saturated fat, 0 mg cholesterol, 3 g fiber, 182 mg sodium

2 Each 2-Decadent-Disk serving (1 cake) has: 203 calories, 7 g protein, 46 g carbohydrates, 2 g fat, 1 g saturated fat, 0 mg cholesterol, 6 g fiber, 364 mg sodium

You save: 293 calories, 33 g fat, 19 g saturated fat

Traditional serving: 496 calories, 6 g protein, 47 g carbohydrates, 35 g fat, 20 g saturated fat, 195 mg cholesterol, 3 g fiber, 369 mg sodium

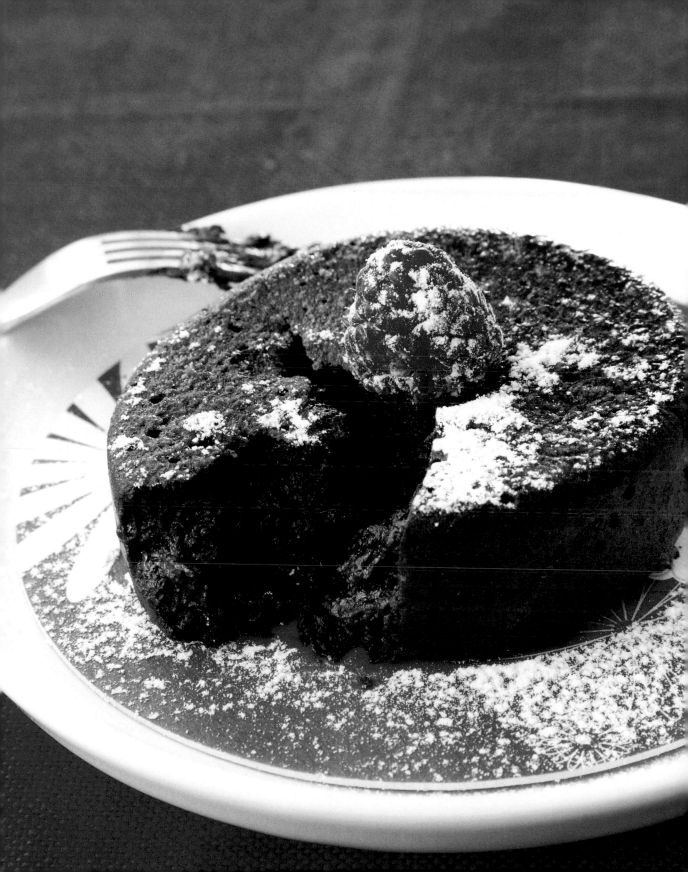

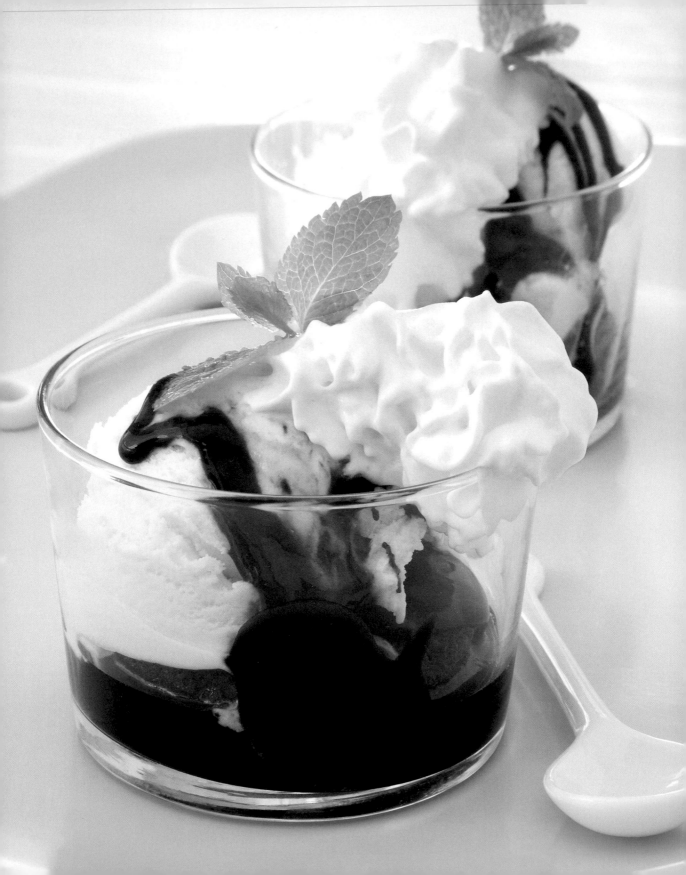

GODIVA BROWNIE SUNDAES

2

I believe that if you put "Godiva" in front of almost anything, it's likely that people will want to eat it. One of my favorite things about this sundae is that it is surprisingly satisfying for only 200 calories. It may seem small, but I've served these repeatedly at dinner parties and even my foodie friends say it's "the perfect amount." And the coolest thing is you can store the brownies in an airtight plastic container in the freezer for weeks (the brownies won't even need defrosting).

I developed this recipe with light, slow-churned ice cream, but I actually love fat-free, too. It's so much better than the standard fat-free ice creams of the past. If you do opt for that, you'll save an additional 10 calories and 3 g of fat.

Butter-flavored cooking spray
2 tablespoons unsweetened applesauce
1/2 teaspoon vanilla extract
2 large egg whites
1/2 cup light or dark brown sugar (unpacked)
2 tablespoons whole-grain oat flour (see page 17)
1/4 cup unsweetened cocoa powder
1/4 teaspoon very finely ground espresso beans
1/4 teaspoon baking powder
1/4 teaspoon salt

2 cups light or fat-free churned vanilla ice cream, divided
12 teaspoons chocolate syrup, divided
12 teaspoons Godiva liqueur or other chocolate-flavored liqueur, divided
6 tablespoons fat-free aerosol whipped topping, divided

Preheat the oven to 350°F.

Lightly mist six 3 1/2-inch-diameter ramekins or ovenproof glass bowls with spray. Place them side by side on a medium baking sheet.

Use a sturdy whisk or spatula to mix the applesauce, vanilla, egg whites, and sugar in a medium mixing bowl until well combined. Add the flour, cocoa powder, espresso, baking powder, and salt. Stir until just combined and no lumps remain. Divide the batter evenly among the ramekins (about 2 heaping tablespoons in each). Bake for 10 to 12 minutes, or until a toothpick inserted in the center comes out dry (a few crumbs are okay).

Transfer the baking sheet to a cooling rack and cool for 5 minutes. Top each brownie with 1/3 cup ice cream. Drizzle 2 teaspoons chocolate syrup over each, followed by 2 teaspoons liqueur, and then top each with 1 tablespoon whipped topping. Serve immediately.

No more than 20 minutes hands-on prep time

MAKES 6 SUNDAES; 6 SERVINGS

2 Each 2-Decadent-Disk serving (1 sundae) has: 210 calories, 5 g protein, 39 g carbohydrates, 3 g fat, 1 g saturated fat, 14 mg cholesterol, <1 g fiber, 178 mg sodium

You save: 117 calories, 11 g fat, 6 g saturated fat

Traditional serving: 325 calories, 5 g protein, 45 g carbohydrates, 14 g fat, 7 g saturated fat, 37 mg cholesterol, 2 g fiber, 211 mg sodium

CHOCOLATE CHOCOLATE BROWNIE CUPS

I showed up to my pitch meeting for this book with brownie batter on my jeans. I have had so much success with these brownies and another variety that I've been making for years that I rarely go anywhere without taking them. I truly believe that in the case of my cooking, tasting is believing.

They're so moist and chocolaty, they often end up on me or even on my publicist's cell phone as we scurry to wrap up pretty platters of them. But we don't mind because they've landed me tons of TV spots and even made this book possible.

I hope you'll enjoy baking them as much as I do and that you'll consider creating your own platters of them to give to people you care about. They're sure to love them and you'll be doing them a huge favor by saving them tons of fat and calories.

Note that they freeze extremely well if you want to keep them on hand for your children's after-school cravings or your midnight sweet tooth. With only 54 calories and less than 1 gram of fat each, you really can't go wrong!

Butter-flavored cooking spray
1/2 cup unsweetened applesauce
1 teaspoon vanilla extract
8 large egg whites

2 cups raw sugar
1/2 cup unbleached all-purpose flour
1 cup unsweetened cocoa powder
2 teaspoons instant espresso powder
1 teaspoon baking powder
1 teaspoon salt
1/2 cup mini semi-sweet chocolate chips

Preheat the oven to 350°F.

Thoroughly mist two 12-cup nonstick mini-muffin tins with spray.

Use a sturdy whisk or spatula to mix the applesauce, vanilla, egg whites, and sugar in a large mixing bowl until well combined. Add the flour, cocoa powder, espresso powder, baking powder, and salt. Stir until just combined and no lumps remain. Working in batches, fill each cup until just barely full. Sprinkle about one-fourth of the chips evenly over the brownies in each of the tins. Bake for 10 to 12 minutes, or until a toothpick inserted in the center comes out dry (a few crumbs are okay).

Transfer the tins to a cooling rack and cool for 5 minutes. Use a butter knife to gently lift the brownies from the muffin tins (if they stick, carefully run the knife around the edge of each cup). Cool on the rack for another 10 minutes. Repeat with the second half of the batter and the remaining chips.

MAKES 48 BROWNIE CUPS; 24 SERVINGS

Each 1-Decadent-Disk serving (2 brownies) has: 109 calories, 2 g protein, 23 g carbohydrates, 1 g fat, <1 g saturated fat, 0 mg cholesterol, trace fiber, 139 mg sodium

You save: 151 calories, 11 g fat, 2 g saturated fat

Traditional serving: 260 calories, 3 g protein, 37 g carbohydrates, 12 g fat, 3 g saturated fat, 15 mg cholesterol, 1 g fiber, 165 mg sodium

"CLEANER" MUD PIE

2

I'm a huge fan of ice cream cakes and ice cream pies for birthdays. You can easily decorate them as you would decorate any traditional birthday cake, and they eliminate the need to eat both cake *and* ice cream. This mud pie is one of my favorites, so I don't reserve it just for birthdays (nor do my dinner guests let me). But by the time you drizzle the warm hot fudge over the top, this easy-as-pie dessert becomes elegant, scrumptious, and particularly decadent.

Butter-flavored cooking spray
1¼ cups finely crushed reduced-fat vanilla wafers (about 30 wafers)
¼ cup unsweetened cocoa powder
¼ cup powdered sugar
3½ tablespoons light butter (stick, not tub), melted
6 cups fat-free churned coffee or cappuccino chocolate chunk ice cream (all but about 1 cup of a 1¾-quart container)
½ cup fat-free hot fudge
12 tablespoons fat-free aerosol whipped topping

Preheat the oven to 350°F.

Mist a 9-inch pie plate with spray.

Mix the vanilla wafers, cocoa powder, and powdered sugar in a medium bowl. Add the butter and use a fork to combine. The crumbs should be just sticking, but not soggy. Spoon the crumb mixture into the pie plate. Use a piece of wax paper to press the crumbs to cover the bottom and the sides of the plate evenly. Bake for 6 to 8 minutes. Place on a baking rack to cool, 15 to 20 minutes.

Remove the ice cream from the freezer to soften. (Allow it to become just slightly softened, but not melted or souplike).

Use an extra-large spoon, spooning small amounts of ice cream at a time, to layer the ice cream into the cooled pie crust, forming an even mound. When the pie plate is full and heaping, smooth the top with a spatula. Return the pie to the freezer for 30 minutes to 1 hour to harden completely. Remove from the freezer.

Put the hot fudge in a small microwave-safe bowl and microwave on low in 15-second intervals, stirring in between, until just hot.

Slice the pie into 12 pieces. Transfer a piece to a plate and spoon 2 teaspoons hot fudge evenly over the top. Add 1 tablespoon whipped topping. Repeat with the remaining slices, or return the remainder of the pie to the freezer until ready to serve.

MAKES 1 PIE; 12 SERVINGS

2 Each 2-Decadent-Disk serving (1 piece) has: 210 calories, 4 g protein, 46 g carbohydrates, 3 g fat, 1 g saturated fat, 5 mg cholesterol, 4 g fiber, 209 mg sodium

You save: 133 calories, 17 g fat, 11 g saturated fat

Traditional serving: 343 calories, 3 g protein, 43 g carbohydrates, 20 g fat, 12 g saturated fat, 49 mg cholesterol, 1 g fiber, 210 mg sodium

EASY AND ENERGIZING CARROT CAKE

2 **3**

When I was in college, one of my best friends, Kier, was mildly obsessed with cream cheese frosting. She would go downstairs to the dining hall every Sunday night to read the menu for the week as soon as it was posted. She'd check to see which nights the dessert included cream cheese frosting (it was usually once a week on either spice cake, carrot cake, or banana cake), and then she'd mark it in her calendar and make sure to be available for dinner. I'd never before met such a pretty, thin girl with such a passion for frosting! With this cake you can indulge your own passion for cream cheese frosting without worry.

Butter-flavored cooking spray
2$\frac{1}{2}$ cups whole-grain oat flour (see page 17)
1 tablespoon ground cinnamon
1 teaspoon baking soda
$\frac{1}{2}$ teaspoon salt
$\frac{1}{2}$ teaspoon ground nutmeg
6 large egg whites
1 cup sugar
1 cup fat-free, artificially sweetened vanilla yogurt
3 cups finely shredded carrots
1 recipe Cream Cheese Frosting (recipe follows)

Preheat the oven to 350°F.

Lightly mist an 11 X 7-inch ovenproof glass baking dish with spray.

Mix the flour, cinnamon, baking soda, salt, and nutmeg in a small mixing bowl.

Use a sturdy whisk or spatula to mix the egg whites, sugar, and yogurt in a medium mixing bowl until well combined. Stir in the flour mixture until the batter is well combined and no lumps remain. Then stir in the carrots until just combined.

Pour the batter into the prepared baking dish. Bake for 30 to 35 minutes, or until a toothpick inserted in the center comes out dry (a few crumbs are okay). Remove the cake from the oven and place it on a cooling rack for about 1 hour.

Meanwhile, prepare the Cream Cheese Frosting.

When the cake is completely cooled, spread the frosting evenly over the top. Cut the cake into 12 or 18 equal pieces. Serve immediately, or refrigerate for up to 3 days.

MAKES 1 CAKE; 12 SERVINGS OR 18 PORTIONS

 Each 2-Decadent-Disk portion ($\frac{1}{18}$ cake) has: 200 calories, 4 g protein, 42 g carbohydrates, 3 g fat, <1 g saturated fat, 4 mg cholesterol, 2 g fiber, 219 mg sodium

3 Each 3-Decadent-Disk serving ($\frac{1}{12}$ cake) has: 299 calories, 6 g protein, 62 g carbohydrates, 4 g fat, 1 g saturated fat, 7 mg cholesterol, 3 g fiber, 328 mg sodium

You save: 284 calories, 32 g fat, 8 g saturated fat

Traditional serving: 583 calories, 5 g protein, 64 g carbohydrates, 36 g fat, 9 g saturated fat, 75 mg cholesterol, 2 g fiber, 335 mg sodium

CREAM CHEESE FROSTING

$1/4$ cup light cream cheese

3 tablespoons light butter (stick, not tub)

1 teaspoon vanilla extract

$1/8$ teaspoon salt

3 cups powdered sugar

$1^1/2$ teaspoons fat-free milk

Put the cream cheese and butter in a medium mixing bowl. Use an electric mixer fitted with beaters to beat until creamy. Beat in the vanilla and salt, followed by the powdered sugar in $1/2$-cup additions. Then beat in the milk and continue beating until all lumps are removed and the frosting is fluffy. Cover the bowl with plastic wrap until ready to ice the cake (must be room temperature to spread).

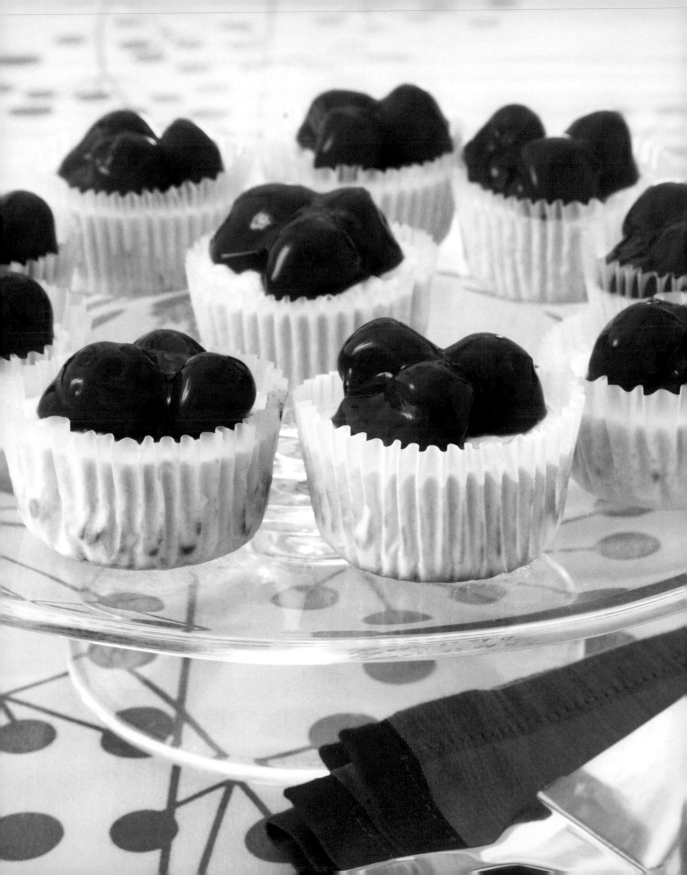

SKINNY-MINI CHERRY-TOPPED CHEESECAKES

This was going to be a recipe for mini-lemon cheesecakes. But when I was making them, my friend Chris popped by and saw the box of vanilla wafers and the cream cheese and said, "No way. Are you making those cherry cheesecakes? My mom used to make them." Then I remembered that my mom used to make them, too, and that so many people served them at their summer picnics.

Not ten minutes later, I got a call from my publicist, Mary. I mentioned them to her, and she had just had one the day before. She immediately said, "You have to make over that recipe." So here it is. If you've never had them and you like cherry pie filling, you're in for a treat.

Please note that when they come out of the oven, the cheesecakes will puff up and there will be tons of cracks in them. This is okay. Once they cool and you put the cherries on top, they will look perfect.

Butter-flavored cooking spray
10 reduced-fat vanilla wafers
12 ounces fat-free cream cheese, room temperature
1/3 cup sugar
2 tablespoons fat-free, artificially sweetened vanilla yogurt
1 1/2 teaspoons vanilla extract

1 teaspoon unbleached all-purpose flour
2 large egg whites
10 tablespoons cherry pie filling

Preheat the oven to 300°F.

Line 10 cups of a standard muffin tin with cupcake liners. Lightly mist them with spray. Place one vanilla wafer, flat side down, in the center of each cup (they will be slightly smaller than the diameter of the cup).

Use an electric mixer fitted with beaters to beat the cream cheese and sugar in a medium mixing bowl until well combined. Add the yogurt, vanilla, and flour and mix on low until just combined (do not overmix).

Use an electric mixer fitted with a whisk to beat the egg whites in a small mixing bowl on high speed until soft peaks form. Use a spatula to gently fold the egg mixture in two additions into the cream cheese mixture until just combined.

Divide the mixture among the muffin cups. Bake for 18 to 20 minutes, or until set (they will puff up and the tops will crack, but this is okay). Transfer the pan to a cooling rack and cool to room temperature, and then refrigerate for at least 5 hours or overnight.

Top each cake with 1 tablespoon cherry pie filling. Serve immediately, or refrigerate.

No more than 20 minutes hands-on prep time

MAKES 10 CHEESECAKES; 10 SERVINGS

Each 1-Decadent-Disk serving (1 cheesecake) has: 99 calories, 6 g protein, 17 g carbohydrates, 1 g fat, trace saturated fat, 3 mg cholesterol, trace fiber, 215 mg sodium

You save: 41 calories, 7 g fat, 5 g saturated fat

Traditional serving: 140 calories, 4 g protein, 16 g carbohydrates, 8 g fat, 5 g saturated fat, 38 mg cholesterol, trace fiber, 300 mg sodium

PUMPKIN PIE BARS

1 **2**

I accidentally managed to include an entire Thanksgiving menu in this book. Though I'm certainly not opposed and folks are constantly asking me for their holiday favorites made over, I didn't set out to do that. According to my friend Kelly, who even owns restaurants and who loves pumpkin pie, these are definitely good enough to serve even at Thanksgiving or anytime. In fact, this is one of those perfect instances where you can serve them and not tell anyone that they're lower in fat or calories. After they rave, you can mention how healthy they are. Your friends might love you even more.

Butter-flavored cooking spray

1¼ cups finely crushed low-fat graham crackers (about 9 whole crackers)

¼ teaspoon ground cinnamon

¼ cup light butter (stick, not tub), melted

4 large egg whites

One 15-ounce can solid pumpkin purée

One 14-ounce can fat-free sweetened condensed milk (not evaporated milk)

1½ teaspoons vanilla extract

2 tablespoons brown sugar (packed)

1¼ teaspoons pumpkin pie spice

12 tablespoons fat-free frozen whipped topping, defrosted

Preheat the oven to 350°F.

Mist an 11 X 7-inch ovenproof glass baking dish with spray.

Mix the graham crackers, cinnamon, and butter in a small mixing bowl until combined. The crumbs should stick together slightly. Transfer them to the baking dish. Use a piece of wax paper about the same size as the bottom of the pan to press them to evenly cover the bottom. Bake for 6 to 8 minutes, or until the crust is slightly browned. Set aside.

Use a sturdy whisk to lightly beat the egg whites in a large bowl. Add the pumpkin and condensed milk and continue mixing. Next, add the vanilla, brown sugar, and pumpkin pie spice. Stir until well combined.

Pour the filling over the crust and bake for 35 to 40 minutes, or until a toothpick inserted in the center comes out dry (crumbs are okay).

Cool the pan on a wire rack for 10 minutes, and then slice into 12 or 24 bars. Transfer 1 bar to a serving dish and top with 1 tablespoon whipped topping, if making 12 full-sized bars, or 1½ teaspoons, if making 24 mini-bars. Repeat with the remaining bars and whipped topping, or refrigerate in an airtight container for up to 3 days.

No more than 20 minutes hands-on prep time

MAKES 12 SERVINGS OR 24 PORTIONS

1 Each 1-Decadent-Disk portion (¹/₂₄ recipe) has: 96 calories, 3 g protein, 18 g carbohydrates, 1 g fat, <1 g saturated fat, 5 mg cholesterol, <1 g fiber, 80 mg sodium

2 Each 2-Decadent-Disk serving (¹/₁₂ recipe) has: 191 calories, 5 g protein, 36 g carbohydrates, 3 g fat, 1 g saturated fat, 9 mg cholesterol, 2 g fiber, 160 mg sodium

You save: 99 calories, 11 g fat, 5 g saturated fat

Traditional serving: 290 calories, 4 g protein, 40 g carbohydrates, 14 g fat, 6 g saturated fat, 63 mg cholesterol, <1 g fiber, 246 mg sodium

ROASTED PINEAPPLE À LA MODE

1 **2**

Though I tend to crave (and indulge in!) chocolate more than any other dessert, I've become a huge fan of this roasted pineapple with or without the ice cream, particularly on cold winter nights. The 200-calorie serving is surprisingly large, buttery, and so satisfying. And if you skip the ice cream, two large pineapple slices have only 117 calories and 3 grams of fat. You're definitely bound to be excited about this way of getting enough fruits in your diet.

If you have one, use a small round cookie cutter to core the pineapple. It makes it a cinch Either way, though, this dessert can be thrown together in minutes.

2 tablespoons light butter (stick, not tub)
Eight $^3/_4$-inch-thick fresh pineapple rings, cored and peeled
2 tablespoons light brown sugar (not packed)
2 cups fat-free double-churned or slow-churned vanilla ice cream

Preheat the oven to 400°F.

Line a large baking sheet with parchment paper.

Put the butter in a small microwave-safe bowl. Microwave on low for 20 to 45 seconds, until melted.

Place the pineapple rings side by side on the prepared baking sheet. Use a pastry brush to brush half of the melted butter evenly over the tops, and then sprinkle evenly with half of the brown sugar. Bake for 9 minutes.

Flip the rings and brush them with the remaining melted butter, and then sprinkle with the remaining brown sugar. Bake for another 9 to 11 minutes, or until the pineapple is golden brown and warmed through. Divide the rings among 4 or 8 dessert plates or bowls. Scoop $^1/_4$ cup ice cream (if making 8 portions) or $^1/_2$ cup (if making 4 servings) on top of each and serve immediately.

Can be made in 30 minutes or less / No more than 20 minutes hands-on prep time

MAKES 4 SERVINGS OR 8 PORTIONS

1 Each 1-Decadent-Disk portion (1 piece with $^1/_4$ cup ice cream) has: 105 calories, 2 g protein, 23 g carbohydrates, 2 g fat, <1 g saturated fat, 4 mg cholesterol, 2 g fiber, 51 mg sodium

2 Each 2-Decadent-Disk serving (2 pieces with $^1/_2$ cup ice cream) has: 210 calories, 4 g protein, 46 g carbohydrates, 3 g fat, 2 g saturated fat, 8 mg cholesterol, 3 g fiber, 102 mg sodium

You save: 161 calories, 18 g fat, 11 g saturated fat

Traditional serving: 371 calories, 2 g protein, 47 g carbohydrates, 21 g fat, 13 g saturated fat, 62 mg cholesterol, 2 g fiber, 151 mg sodium

ON-THE-TERRACE FRUIT SALAD

⭐ 1

I call this "On-the-Terrace" fruit salad because when served in a fancy glass, it reminds me of something that would be served on the terrace at a brunch at an upscale hotel.

People often say that we eat with our eyes before we eat with our mouths, which I find to be true. Simply spooning this fruit salad into an elegant glass instead of an everyday bowl makes it feel more elegant.

That said, I've been eating a version of this fruit salad since I was a kid, so it is very special to me in its own right. Every time we had company, my mom bought a big jar of oranges and grapefruit in juice from the refrigerated section of the grocery store. Then she poured the jar into a giant bowl and had my sister, Leslie, and me help her cut apples, core pineapple, pit cherries, and so forth to add the freshest fruits she could find. She always said that peeling the oranges and grapefruit would otherwise be the most time-consuming part. When we mixed the fruits in the citrus juice, the flavors took on a whole new life, making the fruit salad a bit different from just eating a bowl of apple chunks.

I'm a huge fan of grapefruit, so I use a jar of red grapefruit here, but you could also use regular grapefruit in juice. Though I'd actually prefer to use the unsweetened kind, I haven't been able to find it in jars for years. If you can find it, I recommend using that. Whatever you do, though, steer clear of the ones in syrups. You really don't need the added sugar here.

One 24-ounce jar red grapefruit in slightly sweetened juice or in its own juice (not in syrup)
2 cups bite-sized fresh (not canned) pineapple chunks
1½ cups bite-sized, peeled kiwi chunks
1 cup bite-sized strawberry pieces
1 cup bite-sized cantaloupe chunks
2 cups bite-sized red apple chunks

Pour the jar of grapefruit, juice included, into a large glass or plastic mixing bowl. Add the pineapple, kiwi, strawberries, cantaloupe, and apple. Stir gently to combine. Spoon 1 cup of the fruit along with some of the juice in each of 9 white wine glasses or bowls. Serve immediately, or refrigerate for up to 2 days.

Can be made in 30 minutes or less / No more than 20 minutes hands-on prep time

MAKES ABOUT 9 CUPS; 9 SERVINGS

⭐ 1 Each 1-Decadent-Disk serving (1 cup) has: 97 calories, <1 g protein, 24 g carbohydrates, <1 g fat, trace saturated fat, 0 mg cholesterol, 3 g fiber, 14 mg sodium

PEACH SHORTCAKE

2

Peaches are in season from May to October, so that's the best time to indulge in this dessert. But you can always swap out the peaches for another fresh fruit. About a scant 3 cups of sliced strawberries has about the same number of calories as the peaches here, and you'll be adding 3 to 4 grams of fiber. Or try raspberries; using 3 cups of raspberries will also make this dessert scrumptious. And if fresh fruit is not available, substituting frozen fruit is always an in-a-pinch option.

A lot of people don't eat as much fruit and as many veggies as they should, simply because they say they're expensive and half the time they are mushy, so they get wasted. Well, here are two things to think about. First, when fruit is on sale or less expensive (unless it's on a clearance or bargain table), it's often because it's in season—the crop is rich, so they don't charge as much for it. If the price of peaches has dropped, it's likely to be a month between May and October. Enjoy those then. If the pineapple is really expensive, it probably means it's not in season. So hold off. Second, when you go to the grocery store, ask the produce clerk if you can sample the fruit you're considering buying. Nine times out of ten times they'll let you. Often, after they do, they'll even help you pick the best ones. That way, you'll be looking forward to eating them more often.

6 Better Buttermilk Biscuits (recipe follows)
4 ripe peaches
1 1/2 cups fat-free frozen whipped topping, defrosted, divided

Cut the biscuits in half horizontally. Place the bottom half of each biscuit on a dessert plate.

Peel the peaches and cut them into 1/4-inch-thick half-moons. Divide evenly among the biscuits. Top each with 1/4 cup whipped topping. Then rest the biscuit tops on an angle to one side of each. Serve immediately.

MAKES 6 SHORTCAKES; 6 SERVINGS

2 Each 2-Decadent-Disk serving (1 shortcake) has: 201 calories, 6 g protein, 37 g carbohydrates, 4 g fat, 2 g saturated fat, 18 mg cholesterol, 2 g fiber, 456 mg sodium

You save: 114 calories, 13 g fat, 8 g saturated fat

Traditional serving: 315 calories, 4 g protein, 37 g carbohydrates, 17 g fat, 10 g saturated fat, 104 mg cholesterol, <1 g fiber, 549 mg sodium

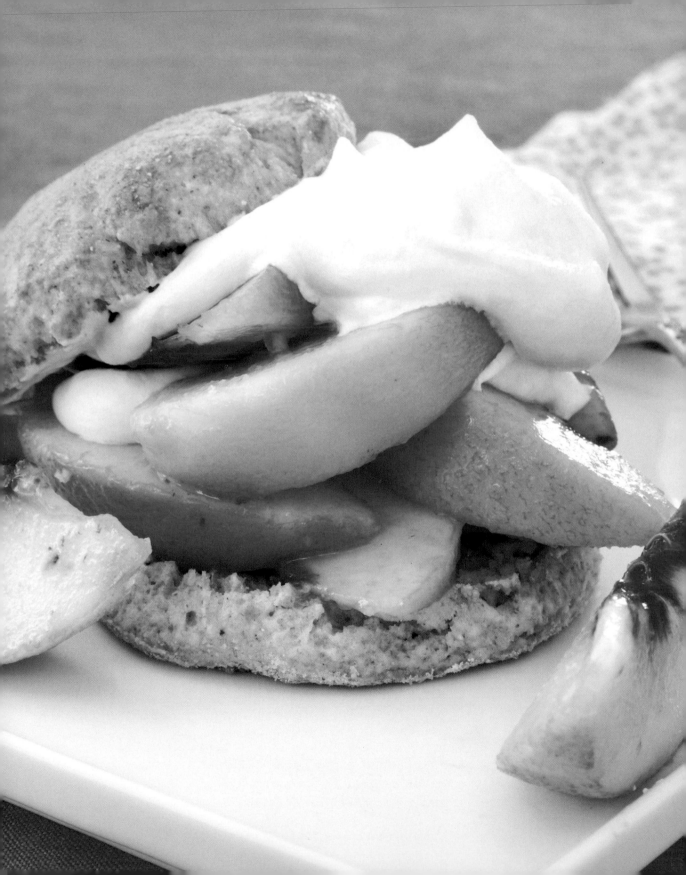

BETTER BUTTERMILK BISCUITS

Butter-flavored cooking spray

$3/4$ cup plus 3 tablespoons unbleached all-purpose flour, plus more for dusting

$1/2$ cup whole-wheat pastry flour

1 teaspoon sugar

1 teaspoon baking powder

$1/2$ teaspoon salt

$1/2$ teaspoon baking soda

3 tablespoons cold light butter (stick, not tub), cut into pieces

$2/3$ cup low-fat buttermilk

1 large egg

Preheat the oven to 400°F.

Lightly mist an 11 X 7-inch ovenproof glass or ceramic baking dish with spray.

Combine the all-purpose flour, pastry flour, sugar, baking powder, salt, and baking soda in a medium mixing bowl. Use a pastry blender or a fork to mix to blend. Cut in the butter with the pastry blender or fork until crumbly. Add the buttermilk. Stir with a fork just until moistened. The dough will be sticky.

Turn the dough onto a lightly floured work surface. Lightly dust your clean hands with flour. Knead gently, adding as little flour as possible, until the dough forms a ball. Pat the ball into a $1/2$-inch-thick rectangle.

Use a floured 3-inch round biscuit cutter or cookie cutter to shape 6 biscuits by cutting 3 or 4 biscuits from the dough. Transfer them to the prepared dish, placing them about $3/4$ inch apart. Press the dough scraps together into another $1/2$-inch-thick rectangle. Cut 1 or 2 biscuits from it and place them on the dish. Reshape any remaining dough to form the last biscuit. (There should be no remaining scraps.) Place it on the dish.

Beat the egg with 1 tablespoon water in a small bowl. Use a pastry brush to lightly brush the top of each biscuit with the egg mixture.

Bake for 13 to 15 minutes, or until lightly golden on top. Cool for a few minutes on a rack.

Makes 6 biscuits; 6 servings

Each biscuit has: 144 calories, 5 g protein, 25 g carbohydrates, 4 g fat, 2 g saturated fat, 15 mg cholesterol, 1 g fiber, 445 mg sodium